T0254013

Parenting Through Cancer

Leonor Rodriguez is a Postdoctoral Researcher at the UNESCO Child and Family Research Centre in the School of Political Science and Sociology at the National University of Ireland, Galway.

Parenting Through Cancer

An Evidence-Based Guide for Healthcare
Professionals Supporting Families

Leonor Rodriguez
UNESCO Child and Family Research Centre, National University of Ireland, Galway

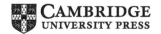

CAMBRIDGE
UNIVERSITY PRESS

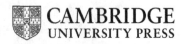

Shaftesbury Road, Cambridge CB2 8EA, United Kingdom

One Liberty Plaza, 20th Floor, New York, NY 10006, USA

477 Williamstown Road, Port Melbourne, VIC 3207, Australia

314–321, 3rd Floor, Plot 3, Splendor Forum, Jasola District Centre, New Delhi – 110025, India

103 Penang Road, #05–06/07, Visioncrest Commercial, Singapore 238467

Cambridge University Press is part of Cambridge University Press & Assessment,
a department of the University of Cambridge.

We share the University's mission to contribute to society through the pursuit of
education, learning and research at the highest international levels of excellence.

www.cambridge.org
Information on this title: www.cambridge.org/9781009009836

DOI: 10.1017/9781009000987

First published 2022

A catalogue record for this publication is available from the British Library.

Library of Congress Cataloging-in-Publication Data
Names: Rodriguez, Leonor, Dr., author.
Title: Parenting through cancer : an evidence-based guide for healthcare
professionals supporting families / Leonor Rodriguez, National University of Ireland,
Galway. Description: Cambridge, United Kingdom ; New York, NY :
Cambridge University Press, 2023. | Includes bibliographical references and index.
Identifiers: LCCN 2022009587 | ISBN 9781009009836 (paperback) |
ISBN 9781009000987 (ebook)
Subjects: LCSH: Cancer – Patients – Family relationships. |
Children of cancer patients – Mental health.
Classification: LCC RC262 .R63 2023 | DDC 362.19699/4–dc23/eng/20220706
LC record available at https://lccn.loc.gov/2022009587

ISBN 978-1-009-00983-6 Paperback

For: Mami, Mari, Olgui and Nina
Y a todos (as) en el Jardín de María

Contents

Tables

Foreword

It could be very easily argued that in order to cope with cancer in your own life or that of someone you love, one must first understand cancer and all its depths, difficulties and nuances. Sadly, very often and for very many, even discussing the topic of cancer in a general light conversation, never mind focusing on its impact on self and others, can be a challenge. While this may or may not be the case for adults, the additional difficulties that arise in the cases of children, youth and their family members in coping with a parent with cancer really complicate and enhance the problem and are at the most personal level.

Thus, this book by Leonor Rodriguez is particularly welcome and timely. As you read through it, you will see the way the author brings a new and very comprehensive understanding to what is known (based on our current knowledge), unknown and subject to other limitations, about the impact of parental cancer on children, young people and families. Utilising research she provides a longitudinal account of the impact of cancer through the differing stages of the illness. The book also contains a very useful description of the role and impact of culture and international contexts of how families experience parental cancer.

One key benefit for me regarding this book is that it is based in the real world of people's lives and experiences. By exploring both the science and knowledge relating to the illness, it also focuses on the issue of social relatedness of humanity and the importance of caring about and caring for those impacted directly and indirectly. The book explores in very pragmatic ways how to support children, young people and families as they strive to cope as well as highlighting existing interventions, which are resources, intended to be of practical help. Importantly the book does not shy away from the 'starkness' of the sadly too frequent outcome of death resulting from the progression of the illness.

One section of the book is fully dedicated to the very sensitive issue of death and bereavement and methods to support children, young people and families who experience parental death from cancer. This is particularly relevant. It focuses on ways for not just surviving the impact of cancer but even ways for those affected to thrive despite it. Towards the end of the book Dr Rodriguez highlights the crucial issue of burden and empathy fatigue, which all too often can take its toll on the carer(s). While personal self-care for practitioners is advocated and the importance of ensuring 'helpers are helped in order to help others' with the risk of burden and burnout rightfully signposted, this is rightfully situated within the wider context of the book.

Importantly for me and hopefully for you, by engaging with the book, one learns so much that is new and contemporary, but the reminder of the importance of valuing crucial support to and from others in coping with parental cancer is really vital. In doing so, one comes to see social support as the 'secret sauce', which enables children, youth and families to keep going. Another crucial benefit of the book is that it is readable for many stakeholders, from children, youth and families to professionals and non-professionals, alike. That is not to suggest in any way that by engaging with the recommended practices contained within the book one loses sight of the person with cancer. On the contrary, I believe this book is both very positive and yet totally sensitive to all the needs of those impacted by parental cancer. This is a right and fitting legacy, which accrues from this book not just for now but for the future.

Pat Dolan
UNESCO Chair Children Youth and Civic Engagement
National University of Ireland, Galway

Introduction

Prelude to This Book

My relationship with cancer began when I was four years of age. I woke up like any other day to go to preschool. My parents weren't there; the lady that minded us was there instead and I remember asking her where my parents were, she did not say. 'They had to go' – she said. Yes, I know that much since they are not here, even at four I could certainly figure that out on my own.

I can't remember my day, probably nothing else seemed unusual about it to me. My mother came to pick me up from preschool and took my sister at the same time. That was weird; my sister and I usually went to my grandmother's house after school, in the school bus. Something was going on. (Routines are important for young children as we will discuss later in this book! And my routine was broken at this stage).

We were brought to my grandmother's house as usual in the afternoon. There were many people in the house. I won't lie and pretend like I remember everything, I don't. I was standing at the main door, facing the living room. I know I was standing on my own. My grandmother was laying on the couch and she screamed and cried in pain like if someone was hurting her. So many people were surrounding her, and it just looked very chaotic and unusual from my point of view. The room was dark, very dark, it was unusual and therefore scary for a four-year-old. I know my mother picked me in her arms and took me out of the situation as fast as she could. I was handed to somebody else and was told not to go into the living room again, as if I was the one who had done something wrong that I was never aware that I did.

My aunt Ana had died, I don't know at what stage I figured that out. I knew she was not in her room anymore; at some point I know I went down the stairs to look for her or just to make sure that she was not there. That was the first time I had 'consciously' heard of death ever before. I did not know what was happening. The distance between the word and the concept when you are four is hard to grasp.

I grew up always knowing that somebody was missing in my life, my aunt Ana. There was a yearly mass to celebrate her life. The first years many people would come, and my family would cook this extravagant amount of food to greet them. Over the years, less and less people showed up. I always knew that people had lovely things to say about her and that never changed so I decided to believe it was true. Cancer took away a wonderful person from me when I was four. I did not know what cancer was for a long time since then. As I grew up, the word cancer became part of language, science classes, other people and that yearly celebration. Cancer took something away from me, something good, and it owed me. All I knew about cancer is it does that, it takes away ... because it can.

I did not know anything about cancer for a long time in my life. My aunt got a 'fright' when I was a teenager, it was just that a 'fright'. The biopsy was negative, but the memories came back to life for all of us. Cancer did not take anything away this time although, genetically, apparently it could. And still can.

At 18 I decided to become a psychologist and then a health psychologist. Cancer was mentioned in the books, and I met a lovely lady that came to my clinic in remission, she had a history of cancer and from time to time the topic would emerge, making me think that cancer really doesn't enjoy just staying as 'history'. She had terrible side effects from the treatment that still impacted her daily life, but the therapy was not centred around that, however, it was ever present. When I got a scholarship for my PhD, I got sent a list of topics, one of which was cancer. I thought that if I was to follow the biggest dream of my life it might as well come with the oldest debt I had as well, cancer took something from me, and I was ready to look at it in the eye and claim back what it took.

Ever since I have been asking cancer so many questions, I do not think that it owes me anything anymore, but it took a long time to convince a four-year-old little girl of that. I do not want any other little four-year-old girl to grow up with that thought, and that has been my mission ever since. Less than a year ago I know the topic emerged in a conversation with my family and even though it has been proven by scientific research that it was the wrong thing to do, my family still thinks that keeping me 'out' of the situation was the best thing they could do. It is not, but I can understand that they had the best intentions, perhaps not enough information to make better and informed decisions and that is what was wrong. I am aware that when I was young, research and knowledge were not as advanced as they are today. So, this is the purpose of this book; this is where it comes from and hopefully what it will achieve. Children and young people should not be 'invisible' or left alone to deal with their own fears and misunderstandings, quite the opposite, children can provide meaning and strength to their parents during cancer, as a crucial part of the care team [1] In this book, cancer will be conceptualised as a family affair, where children and young people are protagonists with their ill parent.

Why This Book?

Cancer is now classified as a chronic illness, due to the advancement in treatment. This means it is important to 'think family' throughout the cancer treatment and beyond [2]. Due to the substantial impact of parental cancer on children and young people, there is a clear need for interventions and clinical practice guidelines to support healthcare services and healthcare professionals to identify vulnerable young people and provide appropriate supports, early and preventative supports [3].

Importantly, research has identified that parents may not be well supported by oncology professionals in how to manage and support their children at a very stressful and challenging time [4, 5]. During illness, particularly during a life-limiting illness like cancer, parents and children need to be supported by professionals involved in their care [6].

It is a fact that offspring of cancer patients may be overlooked by support services as they are not the patients themselves [7]. Young people expressed that they were rarely asked about how they were doing by adults in their lives [8]. Research with children themselves welcomed opportunities to discuss their parent's illness if given the opportunity to do so [6]. It is a fact that good communication between healthcare practitioners and patients can have a positive impact on the psychological adjustment to cancer [6]. Few adolescents, however, had direct access to a nurse or social worker and no adolescents had access to a physician [9]. This finding was supported by survivor research where adults expressed that support for children and grandchildren was not available and was particularly lacking for males [10].

The other purpose of this book is to support professionals, particularly those that are concerned about lacking the skills to support parents and children or may lack the possibility of being formally trained and access further education in this area.

Limitations of This Book

A word of caution about this book is that it is limited by the current knowledge and its own limitations. You will find that most of the knowledge that we currently have about the experience of children, young people and families is mostly portraying Western populations. There is a lack of research with minority cultural or linguistic groups also, including a lack of research on bereavement in non-Western groups and interventions to support offspring available in non-Western populations [3]. Most of the research carried out to date is focused on hospital-based populations, so findings may be limited to this population and not applicable to community-based studies, for example [3].

It has also been suggested (as we will discuss in future chapters) that the gender of the ill parent will have an impact on the cancer experience for patients as well as for their families, children and young people. Most research studies have been carried out with females. As much as 61% of participants are female, therefore less is known about father's experiences with cancer [3].

The research findings are also impacted by who the respondent is. For example, some studies focused on identifying the experiences of children and young people may have used parents as respondents. This may have influenced children's participation and presented the views of parents instead of those of children and young people [11]. This does not mean that all of them were inaccurate; however, to fully understand specific aspects, for example communication, research needs to expand on the respondents that are included, parent–child communication at the time of parental cancer could benefit from including the child and the ill parent's views but also the healthy co-parent [12]. So far, the different perspectives have usually not been included [12]. This would imply more time and more research resources, so there are practical reasons why including several sources of information is not a more common practice; however, the quality of the knowledge generated and made available might be more beneficial and provide a more comprehensive understanding. So, I would encourage it.

The term parental cancer will be used throughout this book to refer to findings of studies that included mothers exclusively, fathers exclusively or a mix of both in their samples. If information is available specifying the gender of the parent, this specification is mentioned and described in the chapters. Some studies report the sex of the ill parent, however, did not include an analysis of the results and findings by sex and this is the reason why the book cannot specify this in more detail.

This book is also attempting to provide a chronological understanding of cancer, which is a risk as cancer may have an unexpected course and sudden changes. It is, however, important to separate results by whether the parent had fully recovered, was still ill or passed away [11]. This is also why a full chapter of this book is also dedicated to approach bereavement separately (Chapter 7).

Another potential limitation of the knowledge included in this book is that research usually includes samples relying on retrospective data which can lead to recollection bias and miss important details of the experience of parental cancer on children and families [7]. Comparisons between studies are challenging as there are inconsistencies in the aspects of psychosocial functioning measured. It was found, for example that about 61 different outcomes and predictor variables have been measured in different studies [3]. Therefore, there is a need to explore the long-term efficacy of interventions and its impact on outcomes across interventions [3]. There is also a need to explore the impact of parental cancer over time and more systematic and targeted interventions that can be used internationally as well as locally to allow for comparisons if suitable [3].

Another possible limitation is the lack of clarity on ages and developmental stages of cancer in the research. Terms such as child and offspring are used interchangeably. Child is used for both under 12-year-olds and under 18-year-olds [3]. Findings for children and young people sometimes are reported together with no clarification of differences between them. Chapter 2 will present the impact of parental cancer by age group, even though the information is limited.

Lastly, in the interest of transparency, I am a psychologist with a background in clinical and health psychology. I have worked with cancer from this point of view but also as part of multidisciplinary teams where, over the years, I have learnt about the medical terms and the medical language, but I am not an expert in the topic. This book is, therefore, focused mainly on a comprehensive understanding of cancer approaching the cultural, psychological, emotional, parenting and overall contexts and experiences of cancer for children, young people and families. This book is not suitable if you are looking for medical expertise. I do not personally have it and I would not attempt to write about it. I hope to share this comprehensive understanding with healthcare professionals and what I hope to achieve with that term is to be as comprehensive as possible. This means to include professionals who might work in the field of cancer, psychologists, social workers, medical doctors, nurses and therapists. I hope this book will be useful to all of you and the children, young people and families who experience cancer that you get to meet.

What Is Included in This Book?

This book includes eight chapters that provide knowledge and skills to healthcare practitioners (mainly) that are in contact or working directly with children, young people and families through an experience of parental cancer. Chapter 1 explores the impact of parental cancer, consciously exploring the knowledge by age group, and taking into consideration what we currently know about how cancer impacts children, young people and families according to their developmental stage. Research has suggested that cancer has different stages and, even though the course of the illness can change, it generally follows identifiable stages: diagnosis, treatment and survivorship. These stages have their own qualities and challenges for families. These will be described in Chapter 2. Chapters 3 and 4 are looking at the context of how culture, policy, socioeconomic backgrounds, parenting culture, parenting practices, religion and other external factors influence and shape the experiences of cancer and cancer care for families. After the impact of cancer and factors affecting that experience are thoroughly explored, Chapters 5 and 6 provide a description of the current available strategies to support children, young people and families, as well as formal interventions available and tested to determine their impact and efficacy. This will help practitioners to acquire more knowledge as well as skills on how to support different families. Chapter 7 is dedicated exclusively to bereavement as the experience of death is unique to some families, not all cancer diagnosis will lead to death, but some will. The needs of these families are unique and therefore healthcare practitioners may need equally specific skills to deal with these situations. It is an additional layer of complexity for a cancer experience, and therefore it is approached in a chapter on its own. The last chapter is focused on the well-being of healthcare practitioners offering some suggestions for self-care which is also a crucial part of being able to properly support children, young people and families who experience parental cancer.

These chapters attempt to be comprehensive and be applicable to as many families and possible experiences of parental cancer. What I would like you to obtain from this book is that every experience is unique, and each family and child will have unique experiences that healthcare practitioners need to empathetically listen to. Healthcare practitioners can have expert knowledge and this book is intended to contribute to that; families are experts in themselves and therefore two experts working together is key to supporting parenting through cancer.

How to Read This Book

Each chapter begins with an introduction of the content that is included in the chapter. Additionally, a summary of important topics in the chapter is included in the 'Chapter Highlights' section. All the chapters have suggested activities for children and families; they are included throughout the chapters, and they could be useful to work with families or to suggest it to families, children and young people to practice together. They may or may not be related to the content of the chapter. Finally, all chapters include a section specifically on the implications for practice that intends to motivate much needed changes to policy and practice that will facilitate and improve the work with children and families but also for you as a healthcare practitioner working in the field of cancer. Most of all, I hope you enjoy this book as much as I enjoyed writing it and learning so much in the process.

Impact of Parental Cancer

1.1 Introduction

I begin this chapter by asking you as a reader to say the word CANCER out loud (or in your head) and write down everything that comes to your mind, thoughts, feelings, memories ... anything at all. It is important to understand what cancer means to you as a healthcare practitioner and remember why you decided to work in the area of cancer, what motivated you to even be reading this book.

The impact of parental cancer on children and young people is associated with the word cancer and what it evokes in them. Family members' initial expectations of the threat of cancer and their anticipatory loss are crucial for their experience [13]. According to research, cancer evokes a variety of emotional and cognitive reactions. Cancer has been associated with death, fear and uncertainty, none of which is a positive concept or emotion. Research specifically on young people identified that death was described as the 'first thought' that entered the minds of young people when they found out about a parental diagnosis [8]. Overall, Visser et al. [14] specified that children's perception of how serious the illness is affected emotional problems more than objective illness characteristics such as type, stage and time since diagnosis. There is still little evidence to suggest that the illness stages of cancer and/or parental treatment determine how children and adolescents function [15]. Chin and Lin [16], for example, found that children in their study were informed about the diagnosis soon after; however, few understood why it happened, which meant that some children thought they were the cause of cancer. Over time, for example at school, children learnt about the causes of cancer including genetics, nutrition and lifestyle.

O'Neill et al. [17] found discrepancies in how the word cancer is perceived by parents, compared with children. Some parents were amazed at how their children adapted to the illness terminology, openly used the word 'cancer' and were able to understand treatments and side effects. When children themselves were asked about the word, they expressed hatred towards the word, feeling scared, shocked, annoyed as well as silly, mean and ridiculous [17]. These discrepancies, overall, support what research has suggested that factual knowledge about cancer is lacking in society and is poorly portrayed in the media [8].

This chapter is focused on exploring the impact of parental cancer on families, children and young people, based on the knowledge currently available, as well as critically exploring the current limitations and areas where more research is required for a more comprehensive understanding of cancer on the family, children and young people. The chapter also shows the variety of effects that parental cancer can have in general, but it is important to consider the individual, their personality, their coping abilities and the context they were living in at the time of parental cancer. This means their experience is unique and should be understood fully as unique, as their own. Young people share some similarities or could share some outcomes in common, but it is important to understand the individuality and provide support to the specific needs and struggles of a particular child or young person.

Chapter Highlights

- Cancer experiences are shaped by children, young people and families' understanding of the illness.
- The impact of parental cancer is varied; the literature has reported mixed findings.
- Cancer research methodologies are different and therefore comparisons between studies and contexts are limited.
- Children and young people are entitled to experience positive outcomes even at a critical time of parental cancer.
- Different factors can also explain differences in outcomes including illness stage, age, sex, coping skills, previous knowledge and relationships with professionals.

1.2   Understanding the Impact of Parental Cancer

Children and young people around the world can be significantly impacted by a diagnosis of parental cancer; however, a major challenge that currently exists is accurately quantifying how many children and young people are affected by parental cancer. Different studies, within the same country and in different ones, include reports of the percentage of patients that have dependent children, which range anywhere between 5% and 30% [18]. Several reasons can explain this difference. One of the reasons is a lack of a systematic approach to quantifying patients accurately and a failure to include information about their family, particularly those who have young children or adolescents. Leedham and Meyerowitz [19] described the children of cancer patients as 'second order patients' due to the impact that parental cancer can have on them, as parental cancer is described as a 'unique stressor' that can lead to a deterioration in their quality of life.

One of the current limitations to comprehensively understanding the impact of parental cancer in children and young people is that research usually presents the effects of parental cancer as two very definite and separate categories. Effects are either positive or negative, but to date the author has not identified a study that is purposefully aimed to understand the effects as a continuum, where children and young people may experience negative, positive and mixed effects of parental cancer in different areas of their lives. This chapter, following the way the evidence is presented currently, includes a separate section for positive and negative outcomes, but proposes that the impact of parental cancer on children and young people should be understood as a continuum that may affect some areas of a child's life differently and this continuum may also be dynamic and change over time.

1.3 Mixed Findings

This section is focused on identifying the impact of parental cancer. From the start it is important to be transparent and the answer is *it depends*. The findings are mixed and there are also several reasons why this is the case. Some studies have even reported mixed findings within the same study. There are also very different outcomes reported across studies, contexts and countries, so comparison can be complex. Another reason for mixed findings is the fact that little evidence exists from a longitudinal perspective. Studies are usually cross-sectional and therefore more clarity on and understanding of the impact over time are needed to be able to better support children and young people.

Walczak et al. [3] reported, for example, that parental cancer may have both a positive and a negative impact on children and young people. Most children who experience parental cancer will show resilience and capacity to cope; however, some will experience separation anxiety, anger, sleep disturbance and low self-esteem [20]. For example, other studies reported only negative outcomes. Altun et al. [21] carried out a study in Turkey to explore the impact of maternal breast cancer on children. It was found that, in comparison with the control group with healthy parents, these children had more behavioural problems, higher levels of attention deficit, hyperactivity and total difficulty scores. Girls in this study also had higher levels of emotional and peer relationship issues than boys and more fear of getting ill themselves [21].

Visible and external cancer symptoms also impact on the way adolescents perceive parental cancer. Lindqvist et al. [22] found that better physical health in the ill parent was associated with more psychological distress in adolescents. There are two explanations of this finding. First, the lack of visible physical symptoms may make adolescents feel insecure about what to expect from the illness. The second explanation provided was that the lack of physical symptoms might mean that families do not acknowledge cancer due to the lack of tangible evidence and, because of this, adolescents are not provided with opportunities to express themselves and deal with their emotions [22]. This is something healthcare practitioners need to be aware of, ensuring opportunities are provided for children and young people to express their emotions and concerns particularly when parents do not have visible or obvious indications of the cancer (scars, hair loss, etc.).

Several reasons have been provided by the literature to help understand these mixed findings:

1. **The informant**. Studies have found differences in the level of distress reported depending on who it is reporting on the child or young person's symptoms, specifically if it is the parents or the children themselves [14, 23]. According to the literature, parents struggle to perceive and report on children's distress regarding both internalising (anxiety/depression) and externalising behaviour (e.g. aggression) as well as emotional and behavioural problems [23]. Watson et al. [24] found that fathers identified lower rates of problems than mothers, suggesting that fathers may be less aware of their children's needs than mothers. However, this study is 15 years old and gender roles in the family may have evolved since then.

2. **Timing**. Differences in the impact and symptoms reported have to do with the timing of when the reports were made (close to diagnosis, months or years after diagnosis) [23]. Longitudinal studies have also been able to identify that those outcomes tend to change over time, for example some studies reported a decrease in adolescents' anxiety and depression over time. This shows that reporting outcomes, in effect, vary depending on when the outcome is measured alongside the development of the illness [23]. Other studies, for example, found that relapse placed additional strain on the family and therefore was also linked to higher levels of unmet needs that may not have been identified at other stages [25].

3. **Age.** Regarding age, findings are mixed. Some studies have described that children's level of experienced emotional distress varies according to their age [23]. Older children have an increased capacity to foresee the potential consequences of cancer and therefore older adolescents seem to experience more externalising problems due to this increased awareness [15, 25]. Other studies, however, have found no evidence to suggest age as a predictive factor of children's adjustment to parental cancer [26]. Some studies also include a very wide age range and use 'children' as an umbrella term. For example, Graungaard et al. [27] evaluated somatic symptoms in children who had a parent with cancer and included 0- to 20-year-olds. This may eliminate the possibility of having a developmental understanding of parental cancer, ignoring the emotional, physical and overall developmental differences that human beings experience at every stage of their life which can impact on how parental cancer may or may not affect them.

4. **Gender of the ill parent**. Differences were identified according to the ill parent's gender. For example, some studies found that girls with ill mothers experienced more anxiety and depression than girls with ill fathers and having an ill father was associated with more unmet needs in young people [23, 25].

5. **Gender of the child.** Studies have identified differences by gender. Adolescent girls have reported more externalising (e.g. aggression) symptoms than boys and higher levels of unmet needs [23, 25]. Other studies have identified that girls showed more internalising problems than boys [15].

6. **Outcome measures**. Comparison across different studies can be difficult, as they all use a different set of measures, even to define concepts such as 'adjustment'; therefore the conceptual understanding of what is being measured impacts on how it is measured and creates differences in the findings. For this reason, aggregations and comparison become more difficult [14, 15, 26, 28]. Another aspect to consider is the sensitivity of the measures to capture the issues that children face when a parent has cancer. Generic measures may be limited [14]. The reliability of self-reported questionnaires has been questioned also. Self-reports have been described as potentially biased and unreliable due to being affected by social desirability, distorted reality, poor recall and denial [29].

7. **Research designs**. Cross-sectional data collection may not capture the full experience of children and young people facing parental cancer [14]. As Watson et al. [24] suggest, it is unlikely that family characteristics are measured before the onset of cancer. Randomised control trials may be needed to further understand family functioning and the impact of interventions as well as more longitudinal designs.

8. **Social desirability**. According to Purc-Stephenson and Lyseng [30] children try to hide their distress, problems and behave better to help their sick parent. This can reduce the reliability of the outcomes identified.

This following section summarises some of the negative and positive outcomes of parental cancer in children and young people identified in the literature.

1.4 Negative Outcomes

Research has identified that parental cancer can have a detrimental effect on the lives of children and young people who experience it. The most challenging aspect is that the list of possible negative outcomes is exhaustive and heterogenous, lacking detail in the characteristics of participants that may have led to these findings and the different qualities that could explain and help to understand the differences identified.

One important aspect to consider is that studies often include concepts without defining them, such as fear or distress. Even though there is a shared 'social' understanding of them, the meaning of these concepts is unclear as is the actual meaning for children [31]. Once again, determining if the same concept was measured across studies is challenging. Additionally, these same concepts are usually measured with different scales; therefore the underlying conceptual definition or theory being measured may vary. The negative outcomes identified in the literature and described below are depression, anxiety, fear, worry, stress, poor family functioning, sadness, loss, isolation, strained relationships, post-traumatic stress disorders and somatic symptoms.

1.4.1 Anxiety and Depression

Depression and anxiety have been identified as outcomes of parental cancer [30]. Wellisch, Ormseth and Arechiga [32] evaluated the emotional symptoms over time of daughters of women with breast cancer. The study found that maternal cancer is not the sole depression causing stressor experienced by daughters. They also experience anxiety in relation to their own risk of having breast cancer, linked also to witnessing their mother's experience.

1.4.2 Fear and Worry

Chin and Lin [16] found children experienced fear of uncertainty because they viewed cancer as a very serious and fatal illness. Fear was often associated with parental death; therefore once young people were assured that their parent was not going to die, this reduced their fear [30, 31, 33]. When a family member had been diagnosed with cancer previously, adolescents experienced more worries and fear regarding the possible loss of their parent [34]. Fear and worry were also associated with watching a previously strong and healthy parent become ill and weak due to the illness and treatment [34]. Even though adolescents experienced fear and worry they often would not disclose these feelings to their parents as they thought they had to protect them [34].

Worry is a common experience for children experiencing parental cancer [30, 34]. Chin and Lin [16] found that worry in children was associated with the impact of parental hospitalisations or medical examinations.

1.4.3 Poor Family Functioning

Cancer has also been associated with poorer family functioning [35]. This will be further explored in Chapter 3.

1.4.4 Stress

Several studies have identified stress as an expected consequence of parental cancer [36] [37]. Importantly, Edwards et al. [35] found that stress responses in children and young people were not linked to parental illness variables (diagnosis, treatment, time since diagnosis) but were linked to family characteristics.

1.4.5 Sadness

Children can experience sadness due to changes in their daily life as a result of parental illness and witnessing changes in the health of their ill parent [36, 38].

1.4.6 Loss and Void

Parental death can generate feelings of loss and void in children, which can remain over time, affecting the lives of children and young people [39].

1.4.7 Concern for Their Own Health

The experience of parental illness and/or death in childhood can lead to health concerns, which can continue over time into adulthood, particularly in those cases where the risk of cancer is associated with genetic inheritance [39].

1.4.8 Relationships

Cancer in childhood can negatively impact on relationships over time. Wong et al. [39] found that adults who had experienced parental cancer as children struggled to trust people and experienced tension in their personal relationships over time.

1.4.9 Isolation

Research has found that children may experience high levels of isolation associated with parental cancer [40]. Children can also experience withdrawal and avoidance [30]. Davey et al. [33] also highlighted that the adolescents in their study felt that they had somebody to talk to about the experience of cancer but still felt isolated: 'unless you have gone through it too, you cannot really understand what it is like to have a mother with breast cancer' (p. 252).

1.4.10 Post-traumatic Stress Disorder

Research has found that members of cancer patients' families may experience symptoms in line with a diagnosis of post-traumatic stress disorder (PTSD) [41]. Parental death from cancer can also be a predictor of PTSD, particularly when it follows a long illness and/or prolonged care [41].

1.4.11 Somatic Symptoms

Graungaard et al. [27] found that children may experience somatic symptoms that can negatively impact on their health, including eating disorders, pain, sleep disturbance and bed wetting. What is critical about this study is that it suggests that lack of information may lead to children over-interpreting or misinterpreting these symptoms. They may not get the appropriate support they need [27].

1.5 Positive Outcomes

Studies have found that children and adolescents experiencing parental cancer may also experience positive outcomes [42]. This, however, does not mean that they are immune or isolated from negative outcomes. Positive emotions, according to Gazendam-Donofrio et al. [43], do not protect children from developing issues, as children are not distressed nor protected by the positive emotions they experience.

Another important aspect to consider is that children and young people may not be aware that they are entitled to feel and experience positive emotions even though their parent is ill. Gazendam-Donofrio et al. [43] consider that children do not comprehend that, despite the circumstances, they can experience positive feelings without feeling guilty. This is important for healthcare practitioners to evaluate if the children and young people they meet may be in this position and communicate with them about this. Some of the positive outcomes identified in the literature and described below are post-traumatic growth, maturity, compassion, empathy, resilience and improved relationships.

1.5.1 Post-traumatic Growth

Post-traumatic growth was described in the study as improved character, greater maturity, more compassion as well as developing stronger relationships within the family [39]. It is a positive change that occurs because of facing challenging life crises. Post-traumatic growth includes a higher appreciation of life, meaningful interpersonal relationships and a higher sense of personal strength [44]. Post-traumatic growth has been identified as a positive outcome in adolescents experiencing parental cancer [7, 44]. Kissil et al. [44] found adolescents have the cognitive ability for post-traumatic growth and to simultaneously process gains and losses experienced because of parental cancer. Wong et al. [39] evaluated post-traumatic growth over time in women and men who had experienced parental cancer and found that the impact of this outcome remains over time.

1.5.2 Maturity

According to Chin and Lin [16] awareness of the fragility of the sick parent and the increased understanding of cancer led to increased maturity, which manifested itself by children behaving themselves, not upsetting their mothers, not fighting with siblings and cultivating a more responsible attitude to schoolwork and household chores.

1.5.3 Future Career Choices

Research has identified that children who have experienced parental cancer choose careers related to cancer to give something back to their community and to other patients [39, 45].

1.5.4 Compassion/Empathy

Compassion and empathy were often used in the literature interchangeably, although they are not theoretically equivalent concepts. Davey et al. [34] identified that children became empathetic towards their sick parent as they had to tolerate the patient's irritability, discomfort or unpredictable behaviour. Jansson and Anderzen-Carlsson [8] found that adolescents had deep compassion for their parent and were sensitive to the feelings of the ill parent. Some adolescents developed caring attitudes towards younger sibling as well. They protected them from worries and comforted them when they were sad [8, 34]. Adolescents also supported their ill parent and families by offering tangible support such as cleaning the home, undertaking errands, ironing clothes, cooking and providing physical care [10, 46]. Adolescents also provided emotional support through prayer, supportive text messages and helping their ill parents with their appearance post treatment [10]. Adolescents also reported being more conscientious and able to support others, such as friends whose parents were diagnosed with cancer [33].

1.5.5   Resilience

Resilience is defined as the process of negotiating, managing and adapting to significant levels of stress and trauma [7]. Resilience in families that experience parental cancer was expressed by having less stress and better communication between them [7].

1.5.6   Improved Relationships

Some young people described how parental cancer had improved family relationships and that they had more appreciation of their families [8]. The impact of cancer on family life is further explored in Chapter 3.

1.6   Factors That Influence the Impact of Parental Cancer

This section includes some of the factors or characteristics that research has identified as having an impact on how parental cancer impacts on children and young people. The factors described in this section include illness stage, gender, developmental stage, age, previous knowledge and coping skills.

1.6.1   Illness Stage

Research has identified some of the outcomes that are expected to happen in children and young people according to the stage of parental illness that they are going through. These vary over time and therefore health practitioners can take this into consideration when working with children and families. The fact that these outcomes are identified corresponding to these stages does not mean that all children and young people will experience them or that they should be left on their own to deal with them. These cancer stages over time are explored in more detail in Chapter 2.

At diagnosis, children and young people may experience different reactions to parental diagnosis [47]. These reactions include emotional upset, shock, tears, fear and anxiety. The time of treatment has been identified as the period where families and children experience the highest need for support [48]. This means that it is a critical time to screen children's distress and provide emotional support if needed [48]. This also means that healthcare professionals should be mindful of the burden of cancer for patients and their families at this time since it is a period of active treatment and possibly close contact with healthcare professionals, patients and families. Surgery, for example, can be upsetting for children and young people. On the one hand, mothers had to be in hospital for several days, separated from their families and disrupting normal routines. If children and young people visit their ill parent in hospital, they might be upset because they are aware that surgery could potentially be fatal. Children could often be scared if they saw their ill parent with tubes or saw blood [47]. Other specific treatments such as chemotherapy can also be difficult for children. Children might struggle with side effects such as hair loss and in one study described this as the worst part of their ill parent's treatment, as this meant their parent looked very different from what they were used to [47].

1.6.2 Sex

Some studies have identified differences by sex[1] (sometimes treated as equivalent to gender, even though these are separate concepts). Morris et al. [7] found that adolescent daughters showed a more proactive approach to coping with parental cancer than sons, and therefore, interventions should be targeted specifically to support sons. Daughters had less open communication styles within their families, and those who also experienced maternal death seemed to have the most negative experiences and benefited less from talking openly in a clinical context. According to the authors these identified differences by the child's sex are important to consider when designing interventions and support for children and young people [32].

The impact of parental cancer varies not only according to the sex of the child or young person but the gender or the sex of the ill parent. Research has found that illness in the mother is associated with more negative effects than illness in the father, suggesting a higher level of stress associated with maternal illness [40]. Some of the reasons provided for this difference include the distribution of family roles, whereby mothers usually have increased responsibilities towards child-related tasks [40]. Since this study was written over 11 years ago, however, gender roles, in some contexts, may have evolved towards a more equal distribution of roles and responsibilities in families.

---

[1] Sex refers to the biological and physical characteristics of a child at birth. Gender encompasses societally assigned roles and a person's identity. Gender is a common term used in research; however, the data is analysed by sex, therefore there is a wide misuse of the term that needs to be amended.

1.6.3 Developmental Approach (Age)

One of the gaps identified in the literature is a developmental understanding of the impact of parental cancer. Therefore, there was an intention to adopt a developmental approach to describe the impact of parental cancer in this book. The lack of clear evidence, however, made this impossible. Most of the literature groups children and adolescents together and makes generalisations for mixed-age groups; therefore the developmental understanding of the impact of parental cancer is still limited. The current knowledge by age group is summarised below with the caveat that it is probably limited and not as comprehensive as it should be to target appropriate support according to children and young peoples' developmental stage. The following section is the best possible description by age group, based on the existing evidence.

1.6.3.1 Young Children (0–5 years)

One of the knowledge deficits in the field of the experiences of children facing parental cancer is the lack of inclusion of very young children. Their experiences are the least known compared with any other age group [26].

Young children can experience distress as they are dependent on the care and guidance of their parents [49]. Separation from a primary caregiver is one of the most significant stressors in children aged 3–5 years. This may be the ill parent or the healthy parent if they are spending time away from the child [50]. Separation can lead to distress responses such as nightmares [50]. Changes in family routine for young children can be hard and distressing [49]. Small children can accept an alternative caregiver if they are prepared early. This means the caregiver needs to show strength, capacity and desire to take care of the children [50] and, preferably, it should be a person they already know and trust. Therefore, preparing parents early in the diagnosis may be useful if they have very young children because they can plan ahead and put in place support for their young children.

Children at this age can easily be impacted by emotional distress in their primary caregiver. It is therefore important to reassure the child that this emotional state is temporary, and that their parent/caregiver remains strong enough to take care of them. Parental emotional distress can frighten young children, who need positive activities to focus on to overcome their fears [50]. Art-based activities, dolls, puppets and fantasy play can be used to explain complex issues to children, for example [50]. Chin and Lin [16] described how young children coped with maternal cancer, in this case, by having a representational replacement, for example a photograph or mimicking their mother's behaviour, particularly when mothers were not physically present.

Children in this age group have no concept of illness and the finality of death, so they believe their parent can return after death. Children are not able to understand the changing capacities of the ill parent because of treatment.

They can repeat a script explaining the situation without understanding it; however, it is still important to let them express themselves and ensure that they are understanding it in very concrete and age-appropriate ways [50]. It is not uncommon that children turn to imaginary companions and use play and fantasy to express their reactions and anxieties. It is important to establish a consistent time in which children can have this opportunity to express themselves, for example at bedtime [50].

1.6.3.2   6- to 8-Year-Olds

Children in this age group have been described as very emotional and possibly blaming themselves for bad things that happen; therefore they should be reassured that parental illness is not their fault [50]. This reassurance from others (parents and teachers), and throughout the illness, supports their self-esteem. Children in this age group also have more advanced language skills, enabling more logical thinking and understanding of cause and effect [50]. They also understand that death is universal and therefore it could happen to them. This can lead to anxiety and fear. If parental death is imminent, then the child should be informed and be given the opportunity for final conversations and expressions of love [50].

Changes in family environment can be especially disturbing for this age group and extended separations from their primary caregiver [50]. Children at this age can benefit from simple, concrete, disease related information (name, progress, symptoms, treatments, causes) [50]. Children should be prepared for hospital visits. They need explanations of what they will see and allow time for absorption afterwards [50]. Healthcare practitioners can have a crucial role in supporting children; however they should also be allowed to make the choice of whether they want this visit or not.

1.6.3.3   9- to 11-Year-Olds

Children in this age group can use logical thinking more and have mastered cause and effect better [50]. According to Christ [50] children in this age group are 'easier' to deal with because they can be provided with adequate and incremental information over time that they can cope with. However, they can become upset if they are not given sufficient and timely information as they might struggle to understand the context fully [50]. Children's questions and observations should be given careful consideration [50]. Health practitioners who are caring for the parent can contribute by talking to the children about the treatment and introduce them to the treatment environment [50]. However, this should be based on their age as well as their own interests.

Semple and McMaughan [20] found that children usually in this age group already have previous experiences with cancer in the family and therefore might have some previous knowledge about cancer which would impact on their thinking and attitudes. Children in this age range were able to articulate the physical side effects of cancer and its treatment including fatigue, pain and nausea. They were also able to describe and perceive the emotional impact of cancer on their parent [20]. Children connected cancer with death and feared their parent would die from it [20]. Children had a level of understanding towards the need for change in family life which was perceived as necessary particularly at the time of treatment and its side effects which had physical consequences for the parent [20].

The impact of parental cancer on school-aged children is varied, some reporting emotional problems while others had similar functioning levels to their peers [14]. Vannatta et al. [51] found no evidence of increased withdrawal or isolation in this age group, nor increased acting out behaviours or changes in prosocial behaviour and leadership in school. It is not uncommon that these children can have bursts of emotion followed by embarrassment or avoidance, as well as experiencing a deterioration in in school grades and interest [50]. Children however need to be given permission to express their feelings freely and be reassured that parental illness is not their fault. Children for example can be encouraged to write about their feelings and experiences as a coping mechanism [50].

1.6.3.4 Young People

One of the first challenges for this age group is defining the limits of their age as a developmental stage. Different sources have used different groupings in cancer research with adolescents experiencing parental cancer. Semple and McCance [52] for example included a group between 12 and 15 years. Huzinga et al., [15] included 12- to 18-year-olds. The World Health Organization has defined adolescents and young adults as between 10 and 24 years of age [7] which is an extensive range; therefore the findings need to be compared with caution as they may not be equivalent.

Adolescents can be at a heightened risk. This heightened risk may be because they have developed abstract and logical thinking that enables them to understand parental illness and its possible complications; however, they lack the experience to know how to deal with it and the potentially strong emotions they experience as a result [50]. Adolescents between the ages of 12 and 14 can become emotionally avoidant, overwhelmed and do not express their emotions openly. This can limit their ability to obtain empathetic support from others [50]. The literature has provided suggestions as to why adolescents may be more vulnerable than younger children. Some of these reasons are:

- Adolescents have more cognitive abilities than school-aged children to foresee the seriousness of a cancer diagnosis [49].

- Developing cognitive and empathetic capacities in young people can lead to more awareness of parental physical and emotional pain [7].

- Adolescents are at a higher risk of having conflicting developmental demands whereby they might be needed at home due to parental cancer at a time when they might want and need more independence. Young people are simultaneously dealing with developmental challenges and demands [7, 49].

Adolescents experiencing parental cancer have specific needs which may be overlooked, and minimal attention is given to their needs. This is due to reduced parental availability and engagement which hinders adolescent development [53]. Other studies have found that adolescents had more emotional problems and stress related symptoms than school-aged children and a comparison norm group [49]. Adolescents reported more emotional problems than school-aged children and adolescence was identified as the most vulnerable developmental stage to experience parental cancer due to a major shift in roles, physical and relational changes as well as their need for independence [14, 36, 54]. Jeppesen et al. [55] found that parental cancer had only a moderate effect on adolescents' quality of life while other adolescents have experienced stress [36].

Young people learn about cancer mainly through their own lived experience and expressed insights that other young people of their same age do not share. This experience made them feel unique [8]. In terms of support, young people tend to look for it in their own social circles, but some did not want to appear vulnerable, and this stopped them from asking for help [8]. Young adolescents may lack support from their peers, as they themselves struggle with strong emotions. However, Christ [50] suggested that adolescents between 15 and 17 years may have a better support network from peers at this age and, therefore, they may be less threatened by the emotional intensity of the situation.

Even if peer relationships are important for this age group, independence was important. Adolescents wanted to handle difficulties on their own and looking after those that were important to them [8]. Some adolescents engaged in caregiving roles voluntarily. Adolescents would also benefit from education, information and debriefing opportunities to prevent them from feeling overwhelmed with the role [50].

The specific topic of unmet needs has been given some attention in adolescent literature. Chan et al. [56] carried out retrospective research with young people between 14 and 24 years of age whose mothers had experienced breast cancer. Distress was associated with unmet needs. About 69% of the sample reported high levels of distress which correlated with high levels of unmet needs including a need for information, practical issues and having enough recreational time. The crucial finding of this study is that the authors described that these needs could be provided for. This means that distress levels in young people could have been reduced or even prevented with the appropriate mechanisms and support. It is not clear from the article why these needs were not attended to, whether there was a lack of support provision, if young people were not aware of the options or did not take advantage of them. Services need to be in place and clear pathways need to exist for young people to make informed decisions of whether they want the support when needed or over time when they are ready to accept help. Levels of distress are reduced over time; however, they remain [56]. A recent study on adolescents' unmet needs further explored the impact of these unmet needs on adolescents [57]. It was found that higher levels of unmet needs were linked with lower health-related quality of life. Higher levels of illness unpredictability were also related to higher levels of unmet needs. These findings however help inform interventions on how to approach these unmet needs [57]:

1. Increase young people's understanding of their parents' cancer and actively involve them through psychoeducational programmes and attending medical appointments for example.

2. Encourage discussion about cancer in the family and encourage young people to attend therapeutic camps (where these are available) as these facilitate skill development and coping with parental cancer.

3. Acceptance and Commitment Therapy can help adolescents with the uncertainty and unpredictability of cancer.

Jeppesen et al. [55] identified some of the needs/wishes of young people experiencing parental cancer. These were:

1. Feeling normal despite the abnormal situation in which they were living.

2. Time to spend with their friends, so they feel heard and understood.

3. Support from other adults such as a neighbours or teachers.

4. Clear guidelines to access support.

5. Be 'seen and heard' [55, p. 52].

It is very important for health practitioners to include young adolescents in understanding the treatment, goals and recovery expectations of their ill parent as well as provide access to education, information and the possibility of talking to physicians and other healthcare practitioners [50], if they wish to. Older adolescents (15–17 years old) may be more emotionally overwhelmed than they seem; therefore assessments for anxiety, depression and destructive behaviours should be in place [50]. Christ [50] also suggests encouraging the expression of emotions through writing, journals, music, art-based activities or socialisation. Some adolescents may also benefit from individual counselling sessions [50].

1.6.4 Previous Knowledge

Previous knowledge and misconceptions about cancer can determine the impact of parental cancer on children. Forest et al. [59] found that children had a knowledge base about cancer before their parent was diagnosed with the illness. This knowledge came from television advertisements, TV programmes and/or awareness of a celebrity being diagnosed with the illness. Children may also have previous experiences of other people in their families or neighbourhoods who were diagnosed with cancer. Science lessons in school were also a source of information about cancer. The impact of this information, however, was varied. Some children were negatively affected if the person had died, whether on television or in real life, but stories of survival provided them with encouragement about survival [58].

Some of the previous ideas about cancer that children may have include [58]:

- Cancer is a common disease: children wonder if they will get the illness themselves.
- Cancer is a very rare disease: some children thought very few people in the world would get cancer.
- Cancer as a disease that kills.
- Cancer is sometimes treatable.
- Cancer as an illness where people lose their hair.
- Cancer is an illness caused by smoking.
- Cancer is a genetic-related disease.
- Cancer is a disease worsened by stress.
- More treatment needed is an indicator of how bad the illness is.
- Stronger cancer treatments mean that it is less likely that the illness will recur.

Children and young people might benefit from discussing with healthcare practitioners their ideas related to cancer and dealing with any misconceptions they may have which could lead to negative outcomes.

1.6.5 Coping

The impact of parental cancer has also been linked with children and young people's coping skills. Coping consists of the cognitive and behavioural efforts to manage an internal or external demand which is perceived as exceeding a person's capacity to deal with it [31]. There are two categories of coping: problem-focused and emotion-focused coping. Problem-focused coping consist of managing or changing the relationship between the person and their environment which is the source of stress. Emotion regulation is focused on controlling stressful emotions. Examples of problem-focused coping included asking questions, reading about the illness, doing household chores and caring for siblings [31]. Refusing to talk or think about parental cancer are examples of emotion-focused coping [31].

Time away was important for adolescents, as it provided them with an opportunity to step away from anything related to cancer and this helped them cope better when things were more difficult [59]. Chin and Lin [16] identified coping strategies used by children, accommodating parental cancer. 'Getting used to it' was described as the 'turning point' that facilitated children's acceptance of parental cancer. Adolescents coped in many ways including religion, prayer, going to religious services, humour, talking 'things out' with others, distraction, thinking positively, keeping active in sport and other activities [33, 59].

1.6.6 Relationship with Professionals

This section describes the relationship with professionals and how this can help children and young people at the time of parental cancer. Professionals include healthcare practitioners as well as others such as teachers.

Literature has identified that the relationship between children and oncology staff may have an impact on the overall experience of children and young people. Children may intentionally have reduced contact with staff as they do not wish to share their feelings with a stranger; however some want direct contact with healthcare staff to learn more about their own mother's treatment regime and prognosis, but not all [47]. Individual differences must be identified and considered.

School can be an important source of support for children, particularly during times of stress [60]. Schools can provide facts about cancer, including statistics, prevalence and incidence, but some of these messages tend to be negative, excluding those of survival and hope [60]. Adolescents going through this experience perceived these facts as depressing [58]. They described teachers as being more interested in knowing how the parent was doing instead of what they were feeling [47]. Azarbarzin et al. [61] reported that adolescents had difficult relationships with their school, claiming their teachers did not understand what they were experiencing.

Hauken et al. (2018) found that children experiencing parental cancer obtained a low score in the school dimension, included in an overall measure of quality of life which indicates significant concerns in relation to school satisfaction and worries about results. According to Aasebo Hauken et al. [62] this highlights the importance of open communication between parents, students and school. Teachers need to have the knowledge and skills to support these children in school settings. Studies also found that there was a lack of communication between cancer-care centres and the school [60]. Adolescents, however, still wanted to be treated the same way as their peers and school staff to respect their personal boundaries [60].

Providing appropriate support, however, can be challenging. Chalmers et al. [60] identified that adolescents said that 'too much' or 'too little' support was not welcomed. Therefore, there is a level of subjectivity, possibly, involved in the type of support and the amount of support adolescents want or need. Another crucial aspect that needs to be considered is families and adolescents' boundaries and privacy wishes [60].

How to play Secret Angels[1] Game [62]

What you do is get everyone together and put everyone's names into a hat or bowl – somewhere that you can mix them all up easily. All you have to do is select a name from the bowl and then you are that person's secret angel and you do good things for them for a set amount of time. It could be a month or a week or longer! You can leave things lying around for them, like nice treats or letters or kind words or flowers, just little things that will make them smile. For example, putting notes in the lunch box, hiding sweets in their coat pockets (p. 9).

---

[1] This is the original name provided for this activity. If the word angel is not compatible with you or the beliefs of a family due to its connotation with religion, it can be changed if the original version is accredited and respected for copyright (e.g. secret best buddy).

1.7   Implications for Practice

- Effective and systematic methods of gathering information are needed to understand the extent of the impact of parental cancer and ensure that service provision is appropriate to the demands and levels of need. This will require the inclusion of evidence of the presence of children in patient records as early as admission into hospital [64].

- Healthcare professionals should support children in developing an understanding of parental cancer [16].

- Interventions should adopt a family-oriented approach where changes in family processes must be acknowledged to improve children and family coping [16].

- There is a need to develop more tailored questionnaires relevant for children and young people experiencing parental cancer [14].

- Research has suggested that there isn't a gold standard regarding who the best informant is. Instead, research findings should be triangulated, including children, parents and significant others such as teachers to obtain a more comprehensive understanding of the impact of parental cancer [14].

- Healthcare professionals need to have a family-oriented focus in their practice but also develop interventions targeted at the whole family and their wider context including school and friends [62].

- Somatic health complaints in children experiencing parental cancer should be taken seriously, particularly by healthcare professionals [27].

Anger Cube [38]

Children draw pictures or write down names of things that make them feel special or happy on each of the six sides of the cube. When the children were experiencing sadness, they could throw the cube and remember their own suggestions to help them overcome their anger.

Table 1.1 is an example of the questions which healthcare practitioners can use with children and young people to explore their experiences [16].

Table 1.1 Questions for children and young people

Dimension	Specific questions
Cancer knowledge	1. How did you learn about your mother's/father's cancer?
	2. Who told you?
	3. What did they tell you?
	4. What do you know about cancer treatment?
	5. What do you think about cancer?
Experienced changes in life	1. How did your life change after the cancer diagnosis?
	2. Have there been any changes in your family's life since the diagnosis?
	3. How do you feel about these changes?
Coping experiences	1. Have you shared your thoughts and feelings with your parents?
	2. Have you shared your thoughts and feelings with your family?
	3. Have you shared your thoughts and feelings with somebody outside your family?
	4. How did you cope with difficult times?
	5. What did you do to make yourself feel better?

2 Illness Stages

2.1 Introduction

This chapter provides a description and proposes an understanding of cancer as a dynamic process of illness that changes over time and brings new demands according to the process and personal evolution of the person diagnosed and their families. Changes in cancer may also depend on how successful cancer treatments are and if they work in the intended way or not. Rolland [13] has highlighted that one of the downfalls of discussions about 'coping with cancer' lies in the failure to appreciate the illness as a dynamic process over time. Each phase of cancer has distinct developmental tasks that demand from families a different set of strengths, attitudes and adaptations [13]. Research has found that illness changes over time, and each of these stages is accompanied by different circumstances and demands [65]. I am aware that what I am saying is worrying for any healthcare practitioner attempting to work in the area of cancer, as it means working with some uncertainty. What follows is a linear guide that may or may not be the course that fits the family you are working with; however, it is important to know and have as much information as possible to make better and more informed decisions. I would suggest that reading the chapter on self-care in this book will also be very helpful if you are struggling in any way now, and the outcome is that families will benefit from your help; what they are going through is extremely hard – be there, do your very best and keep learning.

Chapter Highlights

- Cancer has different stages, and these have their own characteristics and expected reactions in children and young people.
- Current research suggests that cancer has long-term sequels for children and families that could benefit from early intervention but also sustained support over time.
- More knowledge and rigorous research methods are needed to explore the impact of cancer over time on families.
- Fear of recurrence is not uncommon; children and young people will benefit from supports to overcome it.

2.2 Diagnosis

The diagnosis of cancer has been described by the literature as the most challenging phase. This phase, also known as the 'adjustment phase', entails a family's pre-crisis functioning, as well as the presence of protective and risk factors. At this stage, if families evaluate the stressor as normative, they will make minor and short-term adjustments that will probably lead to minor disruption to the family unit [66].

The diagnosis period has been described in different ways by research with young people, including, for example, the use of the terms 'chaos', 'blur' and 'ground zero' [65, p. 109]. Adolescents described that 'time' from that moment was disrupted as they began to live with a high level of uncertainty, impacting on their ability to make plans and forcing them to live in the present [65]. The meaning of time, therefore, was dependent on illness and treatment stages [65]. A cancer diagnosis, independent of its characteristics, is a challenging experience for children and young people. Gazendam-Donofrio et al. [43] suggest that knowing that their parent had cancer had a distressing effect, independent of the details of the diagnosis. Children's emotional reactions did not depend on their parent's type of diagnosis or treatment; knowing they had cancer was the challenge.

Rolland [13] used the term 'crisis' phase to refer to the time of diagnosis and identified some of the tasks that families experience in this stage:

1. Creating a meaning for the illness that includes a sense of mastery.

2. Grieving the loss of the pre-illness identity at a family and individual level.

3. Accepting the potential permanency of the illness.

4. Reorganising the short-term crisis.

5. Developing flexibility in the family due to uncertainty and illness threat.

6. Living with illness symptoms and treatments.

7. Developing a working relationship with health professionals and institutions.

Rolland [13] highlighted the importance of health professionals in this early period when they can influence the family's sense of competence to face the challenges, almost to 'frame' the event for them. He considers that families are vulnerable, and practitioners should be very careful in the messages they convey to families, for example including or excluding a family member (children and young people) from a conversation can be understood as an example of how illness-related communication should be handled in the family [13]. This becomes crucial as previous research in the field has described how young people and parents did not receive adequate information about the illness, prognosis, feelings and reactions [11].

Healthcare professionals need to help families explore their fears and emotions in relation to cancer, evaluate the structural impact of cancer in the family and encourage the adaptation of the family system [67]. Healthcare professionals can carry out specific tasks in this stage to help families, identify their beliefs and shape their coping strategies by exploring families' beliefs about:

1. Keeping normality.
2. Mind and body relationship – control and mastery of both.
3. Meaning associated with the illness by their cultural, ethnic or religious contexts.
4. Assumption about the cause, course and outcome of cancer.
5. Multigenerational aspects that shape the family's health beliefs and responses to health.
6. Anticipate possible challenges and difficulties related to the illness.

Healthcare professionals can build a relationship with children and young people early in parental diagnosis and create a personal contact between a nurse/counsellor to provide psychosocial support in outpatient healthcare; this contact must be maintained throughout the illness [11]. Contact can be maintained through short informal methods, for example, using the Internet, text messages and other means of communication that are friendly for young people [11]. Contact, however, needs at a minimum parental consent and the consent of the young person. Channels used for communication must also be carefully selected to be compliant with local data management law, such as the General Data Protection Regulation (GDPR) in Europe. The ultimate concerns, however, must be safety and for the wishes and needs of children and young people to shape this contact.

The first four months after diagnosis were described as a crucial time for adjustment and the hardest time for young people [34]. This finding is an indication that support provision at this initial stage is crucial [34]. The emotional demand of the diagnosis stage for young people cannot be underestimated when they described that their grieving process began as soon as the diagnosis was confirmed [11]. It is important, however, not to judge the experience of illness based on this period only, as other studies found that emotional reactions at diagnosis do not seem to predict long-term dysfunction [43].

2.3   The Chronic Phase

The adaptation phase occurs after the crisis. It entails the implementation of recovery factors that facilitate the family's adaptation to the illness [66]. This phase, as described by Rolland [13], is the chronic phase that is characterised by constancy, progression and episodes of change. Some of the tasks described in this phase are:

1. Pacing to avoid burnout.
2. Improving family relationships (preventing shame, blame and guilt).
3. Keeping autonomy of all family members.
4. Preserving and redefining individual and family developmental goals.

2.4 Overcoming Cancer

Garrard, Fennell and Wilson [66] describe how families can go 'through the worst of it' and how they identify and appreciate positive gains from the cancer experience, including empathy, independence, closer family relationships and appreciation, as well as more health awareness. Therefore, for some families, not all consequences of cancer are negative; instead, families can manage to achieve a 'new normal' over time. These positive consequences were mostly identified in high-functioning families, and they appear to be a result of successful internal and external resource management [66].

2.5 Over Time

Research has also found that the impact of cancer remains over time, even after the treatment has been completed. Research, however, has suggested that little is known about the long-term impact of parental cancer [68]. Therefore, more robust, longitudinal studies are needed to assess the impact of parental cancer over time [69]. The current knowledge we have is limited.

Bultmann et al. [70] evaluated the quality of life of cancer survivors and their children (aged 6–18 years) and found that cancer had a lasting impact on children's quality of life. The study found that an average of 3.5 years after cancer, children were distressed and developed psychosocial problems that lasted over time. Several years after the diagnosis, the lives of parents and their children could not return to normal [70]. The literature has identified other long-term sequels such as loneliness and distress in the children of cancer patients. One year after parental cancer, symptoms were found in 29% of adolescents [71]. Research with young people who experienced loneliness despite being with others during the experience of parental cancer described that this remained several years on [11]. Opposite to this, Jeppesen et al. [55] found an improvement over time in social relations and networks in adolescents experiencing parental cancer.

Additionally, research with adolescents found that this age group could experience sporadic worries about the recurrence of cancer, even after the sick parent was in remission. Cancer recurrence can have a greater negative effect than primary diagnoses [3]. These resulted in periods of suspicion and hypervigilance regarding their own body [34]. Over time, children also showed concern for their parent's well-being once the active treatment ended [43]. One year after cancer therapy, symptoms in children were still high, particularly showing sleep disturbances and fatigue [71]. Gotze et al. [72] found that children had depressive symptoms beyond patient treatment. This emphasises the need for psycho-oncological support during acute treatment and aftercare for all family members.

From another point of view, Leedham and Meyerowitz [19] found that long-term parental cancer did not seem to place children at a risk of later psychological maladjustment. This finding was true for parents who experienced terminal illness but also less severe illnesses and treatment. Children and young people who experienced parental death were not at a heightened risk of maladjustment [19]. Turner et al. [68], although not solely focused on children and young people, found that family members of long-term cancer survivors (between 5 and 16 years old) had a health status and levels of depression and anxiety that were comparable to the general population in the UK where the study was carried out. A very small minority, however, showed significant levels of anxiety and unmet needs.

Families may need psychosocial and psychoeducational support to help them through a long illness process [13, 69]. The literature suggests that young adults, who experienced parental cancer when young, described that they could look forward and moved on with their life after parental cancer. They even described that the experience of parental cancer enriched their own lives [11].

How to Talk at the Dinner Table [63]

My mum invented this clever game that we can play at the dinner table after we have finished eating. She made lots of cards with different questions on them and put them in a jar, and we pick a question, and all must answer it. It creates brilliant conversations. Here are some of the questions: What does the word success mean to you? What are the qualities that make a good friend? If you had picked your own name, what would it be?

2.6 Implications for Practice

- Take the time to listen to the whole story (beginning, middle and end) with children and families; otherwise, information and opportunities to provide support can be lost [11].

- It would be suitable if an interdisciplinary team could support young people as the diagnosis of parental cancer can have a significant effect on them psychologically. Supports need to be in place early in the illness, irrespective of whether children and families want to avail of them or not.

- Healthcare professionals may need effective skills and mechanisms to identify family members at risk of developing issues in the long term and provide early intervention services that could prevent this from happening or escalating once medical services and cancer supports associated with the treatment have ended [19]. Long-term research has shown that most family members have the capacity to 'move on' in their lives by themselves, but a proportion of them may benefit from additional supports.

- Coordinate appointments for young people to facilitate meetings with a physician, oncologist or geneticist to evaluate the actual risk of them having genetically related cancer, if they wish to find out [65].

How to Make a Vision Board [63]

I love making a vision board. It's a bit like making a positive picture but this time you can include your dreams and goals. It is all about something called positive intention. If you put all your thoughts and energy into something and put pictures up and write down what you want, you can make those things happen in your life. Someone says it's like a magnet, you just have to think about the things you want, and you can attract them to you like a magnet.

To make your vision board, get a piece of strong card and cut out pictures from magazines, old travel brochures and newspapers. Get pictures of what you would like to do as a family and where you would like to be in the future. E.g., pictures of holidays, new activities they want to try (p. 30).

Note: The vision board is more suitable for adolescents. Ensure the vision board includes realistic dreams and goals, particularly when used with bereaved adolescents.

Chapter 3

Parenting Culture and Family Dynamics

3.1 Introduction

The importance of family at the time of parental cancer should not be underestimated; therefore it was deemed that a full chapter should be allocated to parenting and family. Research has suggested that the experiences of children and young people are the result of a function of how families cope with stress rather than a consequence of cancer itself [24]. An important term to consider in this chapter is the meaning of family. Following the definition provided by Hedlund, [53] family should be defined by the person experiencing cancer, who they consider to be family. This may include people who are unrelated by marriage or lineage (friends, same-sex partners, neighbours and members from the extended community). Healthcare practitioners may be in a better position to support patients and their families if they have an openness towards all the possible forms of family.

This chapter proposes that family functioning is a composite concept that includes different aspects, and this means it is even more challenging to evaluate. Family functioning includes attachment, coping, communication and parenting styles. All of this may or may not be impacted or changed by a cancer diagnosis for every family. One of the biggest challenges that health practitioners have is to define what 'normal' or 'appropriate' family functioning is and therefore to determine what is normal and what is not regarding family functioning. A functional family was defined as a flexible, adaptive, cohesive and supportive system where communication is also clear and open [73]. Research focused on the family and cancer seems to suggest that better family functioning correlated positively with adjustment [26] but failed to define what ultimate functioning is or should be. Pedersen and Revenson [36] define high levels of family communication, a family identity not defined by the illness and the redistribution of family roles without impacting negatively on the development of individual members, as markers of positive family functioning. This chapter explores the concept of family and family functioning with its complexities but looking to understand ways in which cancer impacts on both. The chapter uses terminology used to refer to families as rigid, flexible, open, etc. These labels, however, are not necessarily thoroughly defined, explored or even justified. Overall, I encourage healthcare practitioners to get to know each family for who they are, their unique characteristics, away from any labels or unnecessary categorisation. Some family theories have predefined models and categories to try to group as many families as possible in the most inclusive way. Please use these as ways to organise your own knowledge but refrain to apply it in a literal way in your daily interaction with children, young people and families.

As described in previous and following chapters, our knowledge is currently limited, particularly by the lack of longitudinal research which can provide insights on the impact of cancer on the family. There is a lack of evidence regarding the long-term changes of family dynamics and mother–child relationships, as there is a general lack of longitudinal research in the field.

Chapter Highlights

- Cancer diagnosis impacts on families, some are resilient and able to cope, others might experience conflict.
- Family is crucial and it determines the overall experience of parental cancer for children and young people.
- Healthcare practitioners need to get to know families to identify their characteristics, structures and resources to be able to identify needs and meet them effectively.
- Family communication is a crucial determinant of the experience of cancer for families.
- More research is needed on the differences of gender in the ill parent and the impact of cancer on families over time.

3.2 Family Functioning

All families, independent of their structure and functioning, will be impacted by a cancer diagnosis [53]. A cancer diagnosis will destabilise families. Even the most flexible families can find themselves in distress due to changes in plans, feelings of helplessness, loss of control and potentially added economic burden which can decrease the living standards that families are used to [53]. Poor family functioning has been associated with children's emotional and behavioural problems [24, 35]. Every aspect of family life can be disrupted following the diagnosis of a serious illness [6, 74].

Research has defined cancer as a family experience and family members can have as much difficulty in coping as the person diagnosed with the illness [53, 75]. According to Family Systems Theory, the condition experienced by one family member will impact on other family members [26, 65, 73]. For this reason, family members have been described as 'second-order patients' as they have unique needs due to the impact that cancer has on the family [8, p. 397]. Hedlund [53] described that how well a family adapts to cancer is influenced by four elements: family history, history of coping with other traumatic events, communication patterns and family role allocation. So, exploring this topic with families can be useful.

Hedlund [53] described that the cancer diagnosis will impact on the family's ability to adapt, as well as the treatment plan and prognosis. If cancer is considered curable, families will experience treatment, restoration to health and survivorship, but if the cancer is not curable, other challenges such as palliative care and end-of-life supports are required. Therefore, family beliefs should be identified and considered when working with families, as this has an impact on how they respond to the diagnosis [53]. Some families, for example, may believe that if a patient is positive and optimistic, the cancer is cured, so if this doesn't happen, the patient may be blamed and has to carry a huge burden which can be avoided [53].

3.3   Family Characteristics

Research has identified several family characteristics that will shape their experience of having a cancer diagnosis including parental age, the sex of the ill parent, family history, the well-being of other family members and other simultaneous demands. Turner [68] found that parental age has an impact on children's coping. Younger mothers with younger children may experience higher levels of emotional distress. Family cohesiveness has been associated with effective adaptation to a cancer diagnosis [35].

Research found that the well-being of other family members will impact on the family at the time of parental cancer [3]. At the time of parental cancer, family functioning was impacted by the gender of the healthy parent, for example maternal depression was more difficult for the family and challenged functioning more significantly than the ill father's depression [26, 35, 76, 77]. Maternal depression together with poorly defined family roles can also increase internalising problems in children [24].

Previous history with life events impacts on the family's capacity to adjust [53]. Families with previous experiences with cancer may bring beliefs or expectations based on these previous experiences and need more reassurance regarding current treatment, symptoms management and possible side effects [53]. It is also important to find out if families are managing another illness simultaneously (e.g. alcoholism, substance abuse, violence, etc.), as this will significantly increase the burden [53].

Some research exists around specific types of families as well and the impact of cancer over time for these types of families. Garrard, Fennell and Wilson [66] explored the experiences of functioning in rural families. The sample was small (10 families), but the study highlights unique issues and characteristics that these families may experience. The study found challenges in geographical, financial, social and emotional areas. Rural families may have to move or travel to metropolitan areas for medical treatment, and this can lead to financial strains due to accommodation costs, shopping, telephone expenditure, travel costs and reduced or lack of income. Strong family relationships are highly valued by rural families, the impact of cancer can impact these relationships, but they can result in positive and/or negative change [66]. It was also important to preserve activities and routines in children. This became relevant for rural families as they often had to experience separation and travelling to access treatment [66]. Community support was also highly valued by rural families and most families perceived their families as supportive but keeping their privacy was also relevant to them. Support from friends and family was crucial to mitigate several stressors [66]. One of the most relevant findings for health practitioners in this context was the fact that 80% of families included in the study accessed professional support services and described these as valuable and appreciated [66]. This finding suggests that these families may need professional support, and specific supports should be put in place to respond effectively to their needs and characteristics. Therefore, exploring the circumstances of families can be useful to target services more effectively and tackle their specific needs.

3.4 Family Coping

Family's current behaviour and its response to illness is in line with its history of previous coping experiences dealing with stress and illness [13]. This also includes multigenerational coping styles, strengths and vulnerabilities, adaptation, meaning making and identifying any past unresolved issues that impact on the family's capacity to respond to the current illness demands [13, 67].

Research has found that children rely on their parents to maintain the family unit, and parental coping strategies support children in their own coping and wellbeing [69]. Parents are a model of how much children should worry [59]. Therefore, offspring's psychosocial outcomes may be reflective of family coping [3]. Parents who demonstrate coping behaviours can help children and young people cope themselves. Some of these coping behaviours include trying to maintain normalcy, being available for children, inviting children to talk, being aware of the children's behaviour and spending quality time with the children. The impact of parental coping on their children is significant. Parental mood has been identified as a source of positive influence for adolescents, specifically for their self-esteem and emotional-behavioural functioning [78] at the time of parental cancer.

3.5 Family Resilience

Families can find stability and the capacity to maintain a sense of normalcy, sometimes including the incorporation of cancer care into new family traditions, habits and practices [79]. Walsh [80] created the Family Resilience Model. Resilience can be defined as a dynamic process which enables an individual or family to develop adaptive and constructive ways to deal with a critical life event. Family resilience consists of three elements:

1. Individual and family development despite risk factors.

2. Adaptive psychosocial functioning in response to severe stress.

3. Recovery from critical events despite a temporary challenge.

This model of family resilience is made up of nine components [80] described in Table 3.1.

Table 3.1 Model of family resilience

Process		Definitions
Shared belief system: passed on from generation to generation, cultural and spiritual tradition. Determines the perception and reaction of the family in crisis.	Making meaning of adversity	Families see the limitations, suffering in a difficult situation. The crisis is a shared challenge and strengthens family resilience, cohesion. Build a new sense of normality.
	Positive outlook	Hope, optimism, faith, coping, humour and signs of acceptance. Meaning making despite limitations.
	Transcendence and spirituality	Participate in religious or spiritual practices.
Organisational patterns		Families develop new ways of organisation considering past experiences, current relationships, cultural norms and expectations.
Flexibility		Family functioning changes according to needs and requirements of the challenge.
Connectedness		Support, commitment, cooperation and respect between family members.
Social and economic resources		Capacity to mobilise family, social, local and institutional support.
Clarity		Shared understanding in the family about what has happened and having clarity and consistent information.
Open emotional sharing		Facilitate communication of feelings with mutual empathy and tolerance.
Collaborative problem solving		Families have resources, joint decision-making, cooperation, solving conflict and achieving goals together. Past lessons from failures would prevent more problems or additional difficulties.

3.6 Family Conflict

Families can experience difficulties when a family member is diagnosed with cancer. Some of these issues have been defined as poor functioning, strain and conflict. Conflict within the family can happen when the appraisal and coping strategies of a family member are not congruent with other family members, generating stress and dysfunction [36].

Marital and family relationships may also be strained [81] and it can be hard to maintain adequate social supports [3]. Marital distress was identified as leading to emotional difficulties in adolescents experiencing parental cancer [49]. Families may experience conflict due to changes in roles, responsibilities and normal activities [81]. Cancer can also disrupt family life as all members are confronted with emotional, practical and existential issues [82].

Research studies have also reported conflicting findings regarding the impact of cancer on family relationships, while some parents report spending more time with their children and improved relationships after the diagnosis, some parents described deteriorated relationships instead [74]. Therefore, it is important for healthcare practitioners to be aware of potential family conflict, validate it as a normal reaction for a very challenging experience for families and support them or put in place supports for families experiencing conflict at the time of parental cancer, if they wish to address this issue.

3.7 Family Communication

Family communication has been identified as one of the pillars in any research study exploring the impact of parental cancer on the family. Many studies have explored it and all of them agree that it is a determinant factor of how families finally manage to cope with the illness.

Open communication leads to improved family cohesion and reduces psychological distress associated to parental cancer [5, 6]. Effective communication can reduce conflict and role strain while promoting cohesion and mutual support within families [53]. It also enables more effective coping and strengthens the parent–child relationship [83]. Expressing feelings can contribute to well family functioning at the time of parental cancer [11].

Family communication has also been identified as a crucial aspect of children and young people's capacity to cope with parental cancer [84] [15]. Research has concluded that there is a need for honest and open communication between parents and adolescents to reduce worry and anxiety [11]. Children take their cues from their parents regarding the acceptability of communication [50]. Communication between parents and children about cancer is crucial to support children [69]. This communication, however, needs to be age-appropriate and timed to maximise understanding and empathy in the children [69].

Even though open communication is encouraged, this is not always easy to achieve. Huizinga et al. [15], for example described open communication as a challenge because children may not want to upset their parents and vice versa and therefore abstain from communicating openly. Cancer can magnify existing problems and bring additional stress in families with strained communication or conflict in this area [53]. Lack of communication about parental cancer has been associated with increased psychological distress for children, separation anxiety, anger, depression, sleep disturbance, difficulties with school and reduced self-esteem [5, 85]. Shielding children from communication can result in losing the opportunity to enable a child to spend time with their ill parent [84].

Research has identified that women are the ones who usually speak to their children about cancer first. However, some of them waited until after surgery to speak or preferred not to talk at all [47]. Barnes et al. [47] also identified that family discussions may not include the term cancer. Research has also identified some of the reasons why families chose not to communicate about cancer with children [47]. These include:

- Avoidance of children's questions, particularly about death.
- Lack of support from a healthcare professional on how to talk to children.
- Avoiding childhood distress.
- A belief that children do not have the capacity to understand.
- To preserve special family times.

Families who believed in open communication also provided reasons for this:

- Belief in communication and expressing emotions to cope.
- Desire to keep the trust of their children, children had the right to know.
- Open communication can help cope due to awareness of the prognosis.

The literature has also suggested that even if children are not told openly, they still have the capacity to identify changes in their atmosphere at home and in their parent's health [20, 47]. Children noticed differences in parental mood, behaviour, overheard conversations or read hospital correspondence [47]. Since children become more aware of the illness than their parents realise, and lack of open communication can lead to sadness, anxiety, fear associated with misunderstanding, misinterpretation and feelings of isolation, open communication should be encouraged [86].

Parents may also misunderstand or underestimate the children's reaction, also underestimating the children's need for age-appropriate information about the illness and its treatment [47]. Some parents may have perceived that their children were coping well; however, research with children themselves found that they expressed feelings of upset and concern [47]. Semple and McMaughan [20] also found that children can have fears, fantasies and misconceptions about cancer, but this may not be apparent to their parents.

Osborn [28] found that children may hide their emotions from their parents, but it may also be that parental cancer may have limited the opportunities for parents to observe and monitor the children's behaviour. Considering this, the importance of data triangulation is suggested and having consistent methods to aggregate this data is also important [28]. In practice, this means the views of parents and children need to be facilitated and identified as these may not be congruent with each other and children may be needing support but haven't been able to express it with their parents.

Findings regarding family communication are also conflicting, emphasising the need to approach the topic with each family individually and identifying potential needs in this area. Gazendam-Donofrio et al. [43] found that intra-family communication was unaffected by cancer-related stress and parental health status. Overall communication during the first year following diagnosis was like that in families between one and five years after diagnosis, suggesting that everyday parent–child communication is stable regardless of the level of stress a family experiences when a parent has cancer [43]. Overall, it is important for parents to understand cancer communication as an ongoing process (throughout the illness) and not a 'one-time' event [50].

Christ [50] created a typography of family communication patterns which can be useful to identify and understand family communication styles and identify ways to support them. It should be recognised that these are fixed categories which may not be suitable for every family or fit each family perfectly. Healthcare practitioners should apply this model to their own discretion and never replace getting to know the families at an individual level. Christ's typography of family communication is included in Table 3.2

Table 3.2 Typography of family communication

Type	Description
Measured telling	Families describe themselves as honest and outspoken.
	Parents usually took time to process information received and then shared it with others (family members, healthcare professionals). These parents selected the best time to tell their child and kept adolescent children constantly informed but adjusted according to their reaction and information needs.
Skirted telling	This involves talking to children and adolescents about cancer in an ambiguous and indirect manner.
	Information was not withheld; however, the most evocative information was not explored. For example, parents would be honest if the chemotherapy was not working but would not refer to the short-term prognosis as a result. Parents and adolescents would agree that they were on the 'same page', living normally while gradually coming to terms with the loss.

| Matter of fact telling | This was focused on practical issues and not on emotion. It would keep adolescents informed of the illness and prepare for death in case it will happen. |
| Inconsistent telling | Inconsistent communication meant adolescents felt they did not know what was going on. Communication was a mixture of withholding information, delay and then telling very directly. Families in this group usually experienced conflict, estranged relationships, substance abuse and mental/physical conditions such as parental depression. |

Overall, Shands and Marcus Lewis [83] have explained that when parents lack the tools to talk with their children, they are left to wonder silently how their children navigate their illness but do not know what they are really thinking and experiencing. This adds to parental worry, concern and potential feelings of being 'bad' parents [83]. Parents and children are navigating through a 'world of uncertainty' [83].

3.8 Family Structure

Family structure has been identified as a predictor of the impact of cancer on the psychosocial well-being of children, particularly in school-aged children and adolescents that experience parental cancer [15].

The experiences of single parents have been of some interest in research exploring the impact of parental cancer. According to Behar and Marcus Lewis [86], single-parent families who experience parental cancer share the same stressors as two-parent families, however, they have stressors that are unique to them. At the time of diagnosis, single parents, for example may not have co-parenting arrangements in place and may find it difficult to engage someone to fulfil that role at a highly stressful time [86]. This also means that single parents will have to talk to children themselves and generally deal with the children by themselves. Some single parents might also refuse to ask for help as they perceive it as a sign of weakness [86]. Davey et al. [34] found that single mothers in their study tended to hide their feelings from the children to protect them. Children themselves in single-parent households also hid their feelings from their mothers to protect them. Single parents may also experience financial difficulties as they may have to pay for their medical expenses on their own. Some may also lose their ability to work due to illness progression and may also lose their job-related medical insurance [86].

Children and young people of single parents experiencing parental cancer can be afraid and insecure regarding the potential death of their ill parent [86]. Behar and Marcus Lewis [86] suggest that children and adolescents may experience unusually heavy demands for their age, taking over adult responsibilities. What is more critical about these 'parentification' behaviours is that the long-term impact they can have is still unknown by research. When parental death is imminent, single parents may need to arrange custody plans. Behar and Marcus Lewis [86] recommend that children should be included and promptly informed about who would take over parental responsibility. This helps reduce their fear [86]. For these reasons, Behar and Marcus Lewis [86] suggest that single-parent families should be referred to family-centred oncology support services which can make an evaluation of needs early and ongoing.

3.9 Parenting

Research has highlighted the important role of parenting in cancer care, acknowledging this can lead to a reduction in the psychosocial burden of cancer for families [87]. Both ill and well parents, however, face challenges. Parenting issues should be acknowledged as a relevant aspect of cancer care as this can reduce parental stress and psychological distress on the whole family [73]. Poor parenting is associated with poor child outcomes when families are going through a cancer diagnosis [15].

A cancer diagnosis can lead parents to introduce modifications to their values, attitudes and views of parenthood and rearing children [88]. Parents need to protect themselves and simultaneously become ready to take care of their children and a patient who needs to be taken care of [88]. Parents may experience a paradoxical message where they must function normally for the well-being of their children while preparing the children for their death [88]. Parents with small children may be more affected than those with adult children as parents may worry about missing their children growing due to the strain of the illness, resentment and perceived loss [89]. Parents experiencing terminal cancer may feel guilty for bringing children to the world and not being able to watch them grow into adulthood [88].

Another challenge to understand parenting is to consider the differences between mothers and fathers. The experience of ill fathers has not been widely evaluated in research and less is known about their experience than that of mothers [88]. Mothers tend to prioritise the well-being of their children instead of their own while trying to meet the standards of 'good motherhood' [88]. Mothers who undergo treatment for advanced cancer may cut their treatment or adapt their treatments to reduce their time of hospitalisation to avoid being away from their children [86]. Fathers who experience unemployment may find their masculinity and sense of strength diminished as they can no longer provide for their families as they did before the diagnosis [88]. Ernst et al. [48] found differences by gender on the impact of parental cancer, women reported higher levels of anxiety and men higher levels of depression. Men also experienced higher levels of anxiety when they had underaged children [48].

O'Neill et al. [90] explored the impact of cancer on fatherhood identifying that when fathers are faced with cancer, their lives and activities are affected significantly together with negotiations of their parenting role. Rashi et al. [91]

found fathers were concerned with being strong and controlling their emotions. Elmberger et al. [92] identified that mothers, particularly those with small children, were more concerned about motherhood and taking care of their children than about their illness. Some mothers described cancer as an interruption of their motherhood and capacity to care for their children. Mothers in this study felt they were not living to their ideal self-image of motherhood, and this was difficult, they also experienced guilt as children suffered because they were not 'good mothers' [92]. O'Neill et al. [90] have highlighted the need for more cancer research with fathers to further understand their role in children's lives and the impact cancer has on this role.

3.10 Parental Needs

It is also challenging for parents to cope with the cancer diagnosis and the treatment, while they continue to meet the needs of their children [52]. Cancer is usually an unprecedented experience for families and therefore they may lack the experience and skills to cope and properly respond to the children at this time [50]. This may lead parents to experience feelings of guilt for not being a good parent, as parents have high ambitions and expectations of themselves despite the illness. Parenting remains a primary role in women. Tavares et al. [85] found that women prioritised their children's well-being over their treatment requirements.

Research has identified some of the needs parents can have at the time of parental cancer. This information is important to know, as it can be used to identify the needs of parents and respond appropriately to them, as well as be able to find suitable supports for families early in the cancer process. If there was a limitation to consider that this information is usually obtained from cancer survivors evaluating their needs retrospectively instead of at the time, they were experiencing the need, which may have reduced the accuracy of the information. Prevention and early intervention must be encouraged. Parental needs identified in the literature include [17, 20, 48, 85, 91, 93]:

- Need for information about cancer, specifically focused on how to talk to children about cancer and children's emotional reactions.
- Support to talk to children about cancer.
- Protect children from the anxiety and uncertainty created by cancer and its treatment.
- Knowledge about educational and emotional support available for children.
- Brief child- and family-focused interventions within routine cancer care.
- Support dealing with feelings of guilt due to not being able to fulfil their role as parents fully.
- Tangible support from the healthcare systems such as hospital-based transport, childcare services, better access to parking services and access

to home care for patients and their families (e.g. social work, psychology, nursing, childcare).

The well-being of children was parent's priority; however, interpreting children's reactions and needs was challenging [74]. Rashi et al. [91] identified a need of parents to protect their children and keep the equilibrium in their families. To achieve this, parents activate a series of coping mechanisms and strategies:

- Maintain child routines, daily activities (school, bedtime) and daily routines (holidays).
- Selective disclosure. Parents chose to disclose certain type of cancer information only, either simplifying or withholding information, particularly with smaller children.
- Project an image of strength and positivity, which consisted of keeping morale high and encourage children to remain hopeful about the outcome of parental illness. Parents, however, may struggle to hide their emotions.
- Adapting to illness-related physical changes including fatigue, increased infection risk, etc. which impedes parent's daily activities with their children. Children can, however, also support and motivate their parents to overcome the secondary effects of the illness in their bodies.
- Connecting with others in a similar situation provided parents with helpful strategies including parenting advice, sharing tips and recommendations with other parents.
- Seek tangible supports from their social networks including transportation, childcare, preparing meals and psycho-emotional support.

Parents have reported a lack of guidance and support from healthcare professionals. Semple and McCance [52] have highlighted that this issue should not be underestimated due to the compelling evidence that unresolved needs and distress in children and parents can lead to poor adjustment and family dysfunction.

Another challenge regarding parental needs is the discrepancy between the needs of the ill parent and the healthy parent. According to Helseth and Ulfsaet [74], this plurality of needs is a challenge since the sick parent needs to be allowed to be ill and the healthy parent needs energy to care for the family and children. Healthy parents may need to think about other things such as focus on their hobbies to regain the energy needed [74]. The well parent may also experience additional distress related to having to assume roles from the sick parent while continuing to perform their own roles and worry about financial strains, which may also be stressful [89].

Aasebo et al. [62] identified that families living with parental cancer may also lack social support. This is an important finding as network supporters can provide emotional support (being present, talking about the illness, stimulate social contact) as well as instrumental support (such as childcare) and informational support (provide advice). According to Aasebo et al. [62], this need must be approached with a network perspective. The importance of keeping family routines was highlighted by Chin and Lin [16] who identified that children sensed a change in their family and described it as a 'sense of gloom' and 'reduced energy' in their households particularly when mothers were absent due to cancer treatment. Children missed their mother's discipline, cooking and normal routines [16]. Additional sources of support could contribute to keep these routines as well. It is therefore important for healthcare practitioners to inquire about social supports available to families.

How to Have a Special Night [63]

We have a special night in our house, one with our Mum and one with our Dad. It is our special time where we get a whole evening or a couple of hours to choose exactly what we want to do. It is such a brilliant chance to be with Mum and Dad separately and do all the things we love. For example, make dinner together for the family, make treats for everyone, kick a ball in the park, do arts and crafts or watch a film together.

3.11 Implications for Practice

- When a cancer diagnosis is given, healthcare practitioners promptly need to find out if the patient is living with a child or young person, to ensure they are included, and information is provided early on [11].

- Information to children and young people can be provided by healthcare professionals, or another person clearly designated for this [11].

- Helseth and Ulfsaet [74] explained that the needs of children and the challenges of parenting through cancer are rarely addressed in hospital settings.

- Parental guidance programmes need to be introduced in hospital settings to enable parental understanding of the reactions and needs of children and how to meet them as well as the need for emotional support for parents to feel that they can be good parents through their illness as well as aid and support for parents [74].

- Healthcare professionals need education and guidance on how to support children and families dealing with maternal cancer [77].

- It is crucial to support dialogue between parents and their children and adolescents [11].

- Provide information to children, parents and families together can encourage more open communication in the family [11].

- Healthcare practitioners can act as role models for families by creating a 'shared space' where communication and discussions about pain and distress can be shared [68].

- Mechanisms should be in place to screen risk factors early, including evaluating maternal depression and family cohesion, as some families may require supports from oncology staff and mental health practitioners [35].

- Hauken et al. [62] proposed a network perspective was crucial to ensure families have access to the social supports they need. This means healthcare practitioners need to acknowledge the importance of social networks and the benefits of seeking support for families.

Chapter 4

The International and Cultural Context of Cancer

4.1 Introduction

This chapter provides a description of international policy and practice that impacts directly on the provision of cancer care to children and families who experience a cancer diagnosis. This chapter was set out to evaluate the impact of different health systems on cancer care. It was found, however, that little research and evidence exists regarding this topic. This chapter therefore presents examples of international good practice in terms of policy and care, however, not in a comprehensive manner as it was initially intended. Available research is concentrated in certain parts of the world only, limiting access to describe the reality of other areas. This, however, helps to identify a gap in the knowledge in this area that may be relevant to approach in the future.

The response to cancer is impacted by the cultural background of patients and their families [16, 94]. Cultural meanings are associated with a cancer diagnosis and its treatment [95]. According to Colon [96], culture can define how cancer information is received, symptoms are expressed and treatment is provided and accepted, and who provides the care and treatment and patients' rights. It is therefore important to consider the cultural context and its impact on the experiences of children, young people and families when a parent is diagnosed with cancer. Culture in this context is defined as a shared communication system, a shared physical and social environment, shared values, beliefs, and traditions and a shared view of the world [95]. Comparisons between countries, however, are complex since there are methodological variations in the published literature [98].

Cancer disparities are impacted by several different factors including social, economic, cultural and health systems, as illness needs to be understood in the context of human circumstances where it happens [97]. Research has been carried out with some minority groups and how they experience a cancer diagnosis. All people have unique life experiences, made up of cultural, social and spiritual practices, which might be historically related to discrimination, oppression, poverty and exclusion [96]. Social injustice and racism are critical factors in shaping the lives of children and young people [95]. Ethnic minority families have a unique experience regarding health problems. Davey et al. [99]

explained that these families suffer disproportionately from health problems, including breast cancer. Despite this, most of the research has been focused on White and middle-class children [99].

Poverty and social injustice have also been identified as important factors to be considered when evaluating the experience of cancer for families. Freeman [97] explained that the cancer death rate is higher in poorer counties than in more affluent counties. Poverty is associated with lack of resources, information and knowledge, inadequate living conditions, risky behaviours and a reduced access to healthcare [97]. Low-income status can be a significant factor in cancer, as low social class can limit the access to an understanding of interventions available [75]. Importantly, Marshall et al. [75] too consider that cancer can also put families at a risk of low-income status as the financial strain that cancer and its treatment can have on families. Amodio and Roy [100], for example, explored the situation of immigrants, refugees and asylum seekers in the United States. This research found that these three groups experience similar barriers in navigating and accessing the healthcare system, as they experience disparities in incidence, prevalence, mortality and illness burden. Some of the care challenges that these groups face include linguistic barriers, physical and emotional trauma, a foreign environment and reduced access to medical services such as preventative screening in their own countries before arriving in the United States [100]. Additionally, they must deal with a lack of social support and stigma associated with cancer, as well as the fear of deportation and lack of health insurance. These factors may influence their health-seeking behaviours and potentially delay medical intervention at a prevention and early intervention stage, which could have a better prognosis [100]. Parents who received support for their children within three months of the diagnosis experienced more improvements in child outcomes over time [101].

Chapter Highlights

- Cancer research is focused in some areas of the world, more culturally sensitive information is required.
- Data management and databases on cancer need to be improved to determine the real impact and the number of patients and family members affected by cancer.
- Effective cancer care needs to be culturally sensitive.
- Cultural determinants of policy, parenthood, family, socio-economic conditions and family relationships can have impact on the experiences of parental cancer for children and young people.
- Healthcare practitioners can learn and adopt more culturally sensitive practices.

4.2 Examples of Culturally Determined Differences in Cancer Care

This is a comprehensive section of the available knowledge from different countries, particularly focusing on the impact parental cancer has on children, young people and families. One of the main findings of this section is that even in more developed countries, clear guidelines or policies are not in place regarding how to include children and young people in routine cancer care. For example, in a research study carried out in seven countries in Europe, including Austria, Denmark, Finland, Germany, Greece, Romania and Switzerland, it was found that in routine adult care, the mental health of dependent children is not routinely taken into consideration [18]. Another limitation is the lack of databases and systematic ways of collecting realistic data about the number of cancer diagnosis and therefore the number of children and young people impacted by cancer in their parent. Examples were identified from Australia, China, Finland, Iran, Ireland, Japan, Latin America, Malaysia, Norway, Portugal, Puerto Rico, Saudi Arabia, Taiwan, United Kingdom, and the experience of Latin American and African American families in the United States [18].

4.3 Database and Information Management

This section includes countries that have efficient databases to handle cancer information effectively. Australia, for example, has a set of databases where patients diagnosed with cancer can be tracked and their children can also be clearly identified. The Western Australia Cancer Registry (WACR) can link with genealogy databases to retrieve information about children: Australian Data Linkage System (WADLS), Family Connections, Midwives Notification System (MNS) and Birth Registrations. This enables the accurate identification of the number and age of patients and children as well as the most prevalent types of cancer and diagnoses [102]. This can provide accurate information on the incidence and prevalence of parental cancer leading to a better coordination and targeting of services, as well as resource allocation and access to health services based on evidence; however, not all countries around the world have these types of databases and, therefore, the ability to carry out queries between them. Ireland has the National Cancer Registry, which enables the quantification of cancer patients and dependent family members affected by it. O'Neil et al. [38] described that over the past 30 years there has been an increase in cancer prevalence among younger age groups and therefore the chance of them being parents has also increased. According to the National Cancer Registry of Ireland, about 15% of people with cancer are in the range of 20 and 50 years, which means that it is more likely that they will be caring for dependent children [38]. Several countries lack databases and adequate information management. Portugal, for example, registered a total of 33,052 new cases of cancer diagnosed in 2001; however, Portugal lacks up-to-date registries that can provide up-to-date information about cancer incidence in the country; there is instead under-notification of cases [42].

4.4 Cultural Meaning of Cancer

Research has described how cancer is understood in different cultural contexts and how these cultural determinants can be incorporated into routine cancer care. Pui-Yu and Chan [103] explained that Chinese culture is characterised by a holistic system of thought, collectivism, pragmatism and respect for families. Regarding specifically Chinese medicine, it dates to over 2000 years ago and is still relevant in contemporary China. This medicine consists of the balance between yin (softness, stillness, cold and darkness) and yang (hardness, movement, heat and brightness) and illness is defined as an imbalance between Ying and Yang, which traditional medicine needs to heal [103].

Another aspect to consider about Chinese culture is that personal feelings and emotional problems about cancer are not shared openly. Some patients are also hesitant to use the term cancer [103]. Culturally there are also taboos about death which make it difficult for patients and families to engage in discussion about planning and preparation for death with healthcare practitioners [103]. Additionally, Chinese people value social harmony and would avoid the expression of negative feelings. Love, however, is expressed through actions such as preparing meals for the ill person [103].

Due to these principles of Ying and Yang, Pui-Yu and Chan [103] provide several practical recommendations of how traditional Chinese can be incorporated to interventions:

- Incorporate hot and cold meal options in healthcare facilities. For example, hot and cold water as well as microwaves for families to bring traditional food and tonic soup for patients in the hospital.
- Enable a supportive environment for healthcare professionals to discuss culture-specific practices with their patients as well as the possibility of including traditional medicine such as yoga or qigong.
- Due to the communication characteristics described, healthcare professionals should be aware of underlying needs that may not be expressed directly but through non-verbal language or bodily complaints, which are expressions of psychological concerns.
- Families need the reaffirmation that they are carrying out their caring role well and appreciate knowing concrete and specific roles and practical tips (diet, exercise and relaxation techniques) that they can carry out to support their ill family member.
- Interventions and support should have a family orientation.
- Connecting patients with resources and survivors from the same ethnic group would me most helpful.

4.5 The Cultural Meaning of Family[1] and Cancer

Literature has identified how cancer is a significant 'family affair' in some countries and therefore any interventions should take into consideration this cultural factor. If this is not the case, it might lead to unmet needs and have a negative impact on children and young people. In Finland, parental cancer, mental health and family were related. Lindqvist et al. [22] evaluated mental health in adolescents between 11 and 17 years of age experiencing parental cancer. The study found that adolescents and families adjusted well to the illness; however, these families were in an active treatment period and maybe this influenced their level of hope. Overall, the study showed that family is a fundamental part of adolescent mental health at the time of parental cancer. Interventions targeted at improving family communication, problem-solving skills and affective involvement between family members was important [22].

Cancer is the third leading cause of death in Iran. Ghofrani et al. [104] estimated that there are about 84,829 new cases every year, and a significant proportion of these new diagnoses occur at an age where patients have dependent children. In this context, cancer can also be a stressful event which has an impact on the whole family. Azarbarzin et al. [61] explained that family relationships in Iran are very important and that adolescents are more reliant on their parents than in other Western cultures. The study carried out by Ghofrani et al. [104] included young people between the ages of 12 and 24 years and specifically focused on understanding their unmet needs. It was found that these young people had higher levels of unmet needs than other Western populations, particularly in the areas of information, support and healthcare. This was due to the lack of holistic, patient-centred and family-centred care in Iran. Service provision is only focused on patients and does not include their families. Azarbarzin et al. [61] found that Iranian adolescents experienced loneliness, lack of support, depression, lack of protection, disability, nervousness, isolation, stress, fear of parental death, changes in sleeping patterns, changes in appetite and aggression. Findings regarding family relationships were conflicting. For some participants, cancer had a negative effect on family relationships. For others instead, the impact on family relationships was positive [61]. Azarbarzin et al. [61] highlighted the need for supportive educational interventions.

Family has also been identified important in the Latin American region. Finding research studies carried out in Latin America was challenging. The experiences of Latin families have been more widely described in studies carried out with Latin families living in the United States. These research studies are included in this book as these families may share cultural aspects of Latin cultures; however, it must be understood that they are living and experiencing

---

[1] Family may involve ties beyond genetic links characterised by loyalty, reciprocity and solidarity [67].

cancer within another culture and possibly a very different health system. Studies that focused on individual countries in Latin America are scarce. This has some significance as research has found that Latin women tend to be diagnosed at a younger age (less than 50 years) than non-Latin counterparts, which increases the likelihood of women having young and dependent children and young people [105]. Rodriguez-Loyola and Costas-Muniz [67] carried out an evaluation of the challenges in cancer care in the region. Significant findings have been made in the region regarding technology and cancer treatment, which can be compared with international standards [67]. One of the important aspects of cancer care in the region is the culturally determined values, particularly the relevance of family and therefore its involvement in cancer care [67]. Rodriguez-Loyola and Costas-Muniz [67] also found that due to the strong family relationships, a cancer diagnosis has an impact on the patient and the entire family. A cancer diagnosis can strengthen the relationship between couples and increase intimacy, but it can also intensify previously existing conflict leading to separation as healthy partners do not know how to deal emotionally with the situation. Like other regions of the world, the reaction of children and young people can depend on the developmental stage. Adolescents can have a variety of reactions including sadness, anguish, courage and rebellion; but the main one is to fear parental death. Young people can also decide to get actively involved in their parents' illness and normalise the experience.

Rodriguez-Loyola and Costas-Muniz [67] described that family reactions can be very intense and cancer patients may decide to keep their feelings to themselves to appear that they have the situation under control and that they are strong. Latin families are a crucial aspect of treatment by encouraging and consoling cancer patients, acting as a motivation for patients to overcome the illness [67]. Understanding the role of family dynamics in this case can contribute to understanding how to work with patients that might have lost their motivation and could even be depressed. Social support networks, however, need to be educated about the crucial role they have in the cancer patient [67]. Education refers to understanding that patients may need support but also want to be active in decision-making and have the possibility of expressing feelings in a safe space and these will be validated [67]. Another study by Reyes et al. [105] carried out with women below 50 years of age in the US-Mexico border supported some of those findings with Latin women regarding cultural values and family relationships. This study, however, explored the experience of motherhood in this group and found that this was challenging for the overall well-being of cancer survivors, especially women that were younger, closer to the diagnosis, experiencing high levels of stress and those with adolescent children. Mothers described needing to be 'strong' for their children but not knowing how to communicate with them about cancer and being distressed for not being the mothers they were before the diagnosis [105]. Even though parenting was a source of stress, mothers also described their children as a source of strength and support for them. Another addition from this study was the fact that mothers described feeling abandoned and isolated once they completed their treatment. Family and friends who had not experienced cancer themselves also struggled to understand the fear of recurrence [105].

Marin-Chollom [107] carried out a study with Latin adolescents and young people facing parental cancer in their parent in the United States with particular emphasis on the cultural context. This study found that Latino young people face additional challenges during parent cancer such as racism and accultura-tive stress. However, specific values of Latino culture such as familism, spiritu-ality and respect play a crucial role in their ability to adapt to parental cancer. Adolescents with a higher endorsement of these values experienced lower levels of depression and anxiety and more control.

Another country context in which family is very important and, therefore, impacts on the cancer experience is Malaysia. Ainuddin et al. [108] identified that family members in Malaysia are affected by the diagnosis of cancer in another family member. A cancer diagnosis can generate trauma, disturbed lifestyle and financial demands which can impact negatively on the well-being of family members. This is heightened by the fact that a cancer diagnosis in Malaysia is usually given at a very late stage of the disease. Saat, Hepworth and Jackson [109] identified that Malay children can adopt a caring role when their parent is diag-nosed with cancer. Older child carers had information and managed to explain cancer using medical terminology [109]. Adolescents living with a parent with cancer showed poor emotional functioning, sadness, fear, sleep disturbances, anger and anxiety, particularly female adolescents [106]. The negative impact of parental cancer on adolescents' quality of life was manifested in adolescents' school functioning and emotional functioning [108]. In this context also, infor-mation provided to children was usually based on parental views of those per-ceived information needs, not on the empirical proof of children's actual needs and experiences, even though the study included children between the ages of 6 and 18 years [109]. The findings of this study therefore may suggest a passive role of children and young people in terms of their capacity to express their needs or the culturally acceptable opportunities given for them to do so.

Research carried out with African American adolescents provides evi-dence of how cultural factors can impact on people's experience of parental cancer. African American families are more likely to develop cancer than other racial or ethnic groups; additionally, they have a lower relative five-year sur-vival rate compared to Caucasian groups [110]. Davey et al. [99] described that African American adolescents deal with normal developmental challenges but also experience additional stressors such as poverty and racism. Davey et al. [99] also found that for these adolescents, avoidance and distraction helped them have a sense of normality and take a 'break from cancer'. Contrary to Caucasian samples, African American families have a strong support system including nuclear and extended family, which helped them cope with parental cancer. Despite this, some adolescents still felt overlooked and unappreciated [99]. Praying was also described as an important family routine and a way of bonding with the ill parent by praying together [99]. Overall, Davey et al. [33] identified differences that they associated with race. According to this research, adolescents are more private with their feelings and did not share them with their mothers in order to protect them.

4.6 Legal and Policy Guidelines for Children and Young People

In most countries, there are no policies or guidelines targeted at supporting children and young people who experience parental cancer except in Nordic countries including Norway and Sweden. The first example of this good practice is taken from the Swedish model of care. This country has made policy changes to ensure the rights of children when their parents are ill. In 2010, an addendum was added to the 'Health and Medicine Services Act' where it is now stated that it is the responsibility of healthcare professionals to consider children's needs for information advice and support. This is clearly a very important advance in terms of policy; however, giving this responsibility solely to healthcare professionals may not be realistic and a big additional burden on professionals. Research has advocated for a coordinated and interdisciplinary approach to cancer care [109].

Chapter 5, Section 7 states that [111]:

A child's need for information, advice and support shall be taken into account in particular if the child's parent or any other adult with whom the child resides permanently with 1. has a mental disorder or a mental disability, 2. have a serious physical illness or injury, or 3. have an addiction to alcohol, other addictive agents or gambling.

The same applies if the child's parent or any other adult with whom the child lives permanently dies unexpectedly. *Law (2017:810).* (Health Care Act (2017:30) Swedish Constitution Collection 2017:2017:30 t.o.m. SFS 2021:648 - Riksdag (riksdagen.se)

Norway is denominated as a welfare state; this means that cancer care is available to all for free. Cancer patients can also have access to multiple welfare benefits that support the loss in earnings, for example [113]. In Norway, healthcare professionals are legally bound by 'The Act on Health Personnel' to focus on children's well-being when a parent is ill. Oncology Departments must assign a healthcare practitioner to document the experiences of minor children and ensure they are involved in assessments. This practitioner is also obliged to contact social services, if necessary, without having to seek parental consent [113]. Despite this, a study carried out by Hauken et al. [62] found that compared to the norm, children living with a parent diagnosed with cancer scored significantly higher in levels of anxiety but not in their levels of worry and concentration. This was particularly the case for older children. Children scored lower in physical, emotional well-being and school. Similar scores were identified in the intervention and the control group in their quality of life, self-esteem, family and friend dimensions [62].

Niemela et al. [71] investigated psychiatric diagnoses given to children impacted by parental cancer in psychiatric and somatic healthcare settings in Finland. The study found that daughters of a parent with cancer are more likely to require outpatient treatment for mental health disorders than peers. The study, however, did not find evidence of children experiencing more hospital-treated psychiatric disorders associated with parental cancer. The study overall associates referral to specialised psychiatric outpatient clinics with parental cancer [71].

Other countries have made advancements towards achieving these guidelines and policies. For example, the National Institute for Health Care Excellence (NICE) in the United Kingdom provides evidence-based recommendations for health and care, illness preventions, and improving health and care services. NICE Guidelines in the United Kingdom have advocated since 2004 for the inclusion of psychological support for families of patients. Although this is an important policy advancement, research has pointed out that there are no clear guidelines on how services can best respond to the unmet needs of children and families, and these may go unnoticed [24].

4.7 The Impact of Cancer on Children and Young People

This section has described the impact of cancer specifically on children and young people in different countries of the world. It is important to remember that different cultural contexts might have a different effect on the experience of children and young people but also these studies measured different outcomes and therefore comparison between them was not intended and therefore not possible. For example, Costas-Muniz [106] carried out a study with Puerto Rican young people. It was found that these young people mostly used positive methods and emotion-focused coping strategies to deal with their difficulties, including acceptance, seeking emotional support and religion. The study identified, however, that 64% of these young people had clinical levels of depression and 44% had elevated levels of anxiety, associated with coping strategies such as denial, behavioural disengagement and acceptance. Denial, in this case, led to more distress as it can be an attempt to avoid dealing with the stressful events. This study, however, makes no reference to the cultural or medical context of these young people. It only suggests that the sample size was small based on cross-sectional data. The impact of cancer on young people was also described in Saudi Arabia. In this country, breast cancer has been described as a 'major health problem' that affects both women and their families [114]. An important challenge in Saudi Arabia is that talking about cancer is still considered a sensitive issue to discuss with school-aged children. Parents are usually expected to make a judgement on how best to achieve this with little guidance on how to do it. The study by Al-Zaben et al. [114] found that in those cases where mothers spoke with their children about maternal cancer, over 80% of children showed improvements in the way they acted, and the mother-child relationship also improved. There was, however, a negative impact on school performance identified in 77% of children included in the study. Al-Zaben et al. [114] explained this finding as attention being diverted away from school to more important issues such as family relationships, given that culturally family is very important. This was, however, a small study with a convenience sample, therefore, the findings may not be generalisable to all the country. The study shows that findings from Western countries may not be applicable to women and families from this part of the world and cultural differences need to be considered when understanding the experience of cancer for families in Saudi Arabia.

Chin and Lin [16] carried out a study with children in Taiwan and identified the culturally dependent factors that determine children and family coping. Children in this study usually learnt about cancer diagnosis from their mothers and this seems to be a female role as fathers are described as having an 'absent present' father role, meaning they had an overall weak role in family communication. According to Chin and Lin [16], Taiwanese fathers are the 'masters' in the family and are the economic providers, whereas domestic affairs are female's business. Other children described that the information they obtained came from overhearing parental conversations, and therefore cancer communication was restricted. According to Chin and Lin [16], Taiwanese children experienced an array of emotions including shock, sadness, worry and fear. Like Western cultures, the difference was that they tend to keep their worries and fears to themselves. Family communication was also culturally determined. Children did not express their worries and fear to family members due to personal characteristics of the child (shyness), but it was mostly compliant with a maternal request for secrecy regarding their diagnosis. Chang [115] identified a similar situation in the other direction, meaning that mothers had discussions with their daughters, but these did not include any emotional content to avoid personal topics as this could negatively influence their daughter's moods and emotions. According to Chang [115], mothers in Taiwanese culture are expected to ensure that their children are nurtured, well, healthy and successful. Having a cancer diagnosis, breast cancer specifically, means that a mother has failed at her role and can negatively impact their children's current and future enrolment in school or in the workplace.

According to Chin and Lin [16], there is also a culturally determined desire for secrecy as people are concerned about others' judgements and therefore do not disclose their problems publicly. Some children also expressed that they expected minimising responses, protective lies or preaching and therefore decided against expressing their opinions. According to Chin and Lin [16], Asian family structures are vertical, which means parents tend to instruct and lecture, discouraging children from expressing their emotions and opinions. Communication with siblings was also limited, some children described disinterest, children being too young to understand, avoid upsetting them or not having a close relationship with them. Caring roles in children, like the case described in Malaysia, were also significant in this study. Chin and Lin [16] found that school-aged children were sensitive to their mother's condition, became aware of the importance of self-regulation and became protective in the mother–child relationship. Preadolescent girls engaged in consoling and nurturing behaviour with their mothers, initiating a pep talk, provided emotional care and avoided irritating their mothers. Due to the high value of academic success in Asian cultures, children would also engage in getting good grades to reduce maternal worry.

In the continent of Africa, on a study carried out in Tunisia, Korbi et al. [116] found that 96% of parents in their study reported behavioural changes including anxiety, depression, violent behaviour and aggression, emotional dependency and addiction. Overall, Tunisian parents involve their children in the disease despite the developmental disruption it may lead to. Younger children, in preschool age, were less aware of parental cancer as parents were in fear of generating emotional and behavioural trauma in them.

4.8 Parenthood Culture and Its Impact on Cancer

In some cultures, culturally defined parenthood practices can have an impact on the cancer experience. Inoue et al. [117] carried out a national profile impacted by parental cancer in Japan. The authors identified an important demographic characteristic which is impacting the experience of parental cancer. As couples are postponing parenthood, this increases the probability that they will experience cancer while having a young dependent child, who can experience higher levels of stress due to parental illness/death. The study showed that of the annual diagnoses of cancer in adults in a year, 56,143 were parents, which meant that 87,017 children experienced the impact of parental cancer in a year. This estimation, however, can be an underestimation as providing information to the Japanese population-based cancer registry is not compulsory.

4.9 Recommendations to Increase Cultural Sensitivity

- **Language barriers**. Practitioners can help overcome language barriers. Having bilingual and bicultural staff can help but also the use of professional interpreters rather than family members to translate is important [96].

- **Visual aids**. Using visual aids instead of only text-based information can help patients increase their understanding of their own diagnosis and treatment [96].

- **Awareness**. Practitioners need to be aware that their own cultural beliefs and biases may have an impact on the care of the patient. Practitioners need to actively explore the differences they bring to the interactions with their patients [96].

How to say Thank You [63]

This is a really easy thing to do that can make you see all good things that have happened in your day, which you might not have even noticed. Keep a positive diary and write down five good things about yourself or things that you have done well or things that have happened to you. Some days it is easier to do so than others. If you have a good day, you might be able to write down even more than five. If you have had a bad day, you might not want to write anything, but you have to try! The more you do it, the easier it will be to focus on good and positive things (p. 40)

4.10 Implications for Practice

- Specific geographical areas, particularly those with higher cancer mortality rates, should be identified and targeted with culturally relevant education, access to screening, treatment and diagnosis as well as improved social support [97]. All these factors will help reduce culturally and socially determined inequalities in cancer. (I am very aware that this needs resources and possibly many; however, it is important to strive and improve cancer care all over the world.)

- There is currently a need for intervention models that consider the differences in culture and socio-economic backgrounds, as these are crucial to understand how families experience a cancer diagnosis [75].

- Some of the elements that culturally sensitive interventions should consider are flexibility (schedule interventions according to work and other family requirements), language (conducting interventions in other languages), travel (bring interventions to local places and health clinics), financial concerns (include information about financial resources available), child and family environments (provide childcare and food to ensure families can attend sessions) and include follow-up and referrals to community agencies for additional supports [75].

- Learning about culture can help healthcare practitioners provide culturally sensitive and psychosocial interventions to patients and families during cancer care [96]. According to Colon [96], making assumptions about the culture of a patient can impact negatively on the provision of culturally sensitive interventions [96].

- Due to potential cultural differences, it is essential for healthcare practitioners to learn to work with resistance patiently, particularly with older and more traditional patients and their families [103].

- More education for physicians, patients and families should be provided so that they can understand the value and needs for connecting survivors to reduce fear, isolation and improve the quality of survivorship [105]. Ideally these support spaces may benefit from being culturally conscious, engaging but also supporting patients and families in spaces where they feel comfortable [105].

Supporting Children and Young People Through Parental Cancer

5.1 Introduction

This book is openly in favour of involving children and young people in parental cancer; it will build a case based on the current evidence that is best to communicate with and involve them honestly, as early as possible. Involving children and young people is still a challenge and a responsibility from the adult in the relationship, the parent and the healthcare practitioner. Children and young people should only be involved if the appropriate conditions are in place to ensure their safety. Another important and probably the most important aspect to consider is their wishes; children and young people are entitled to be involved according to their needs, wishes and capacities on when and how they can and want to be engaged. I am also aware that in some circumstances, children may have conditions or circumstances of their own which means that for their own well-being, protecting them from parental cancer may be instead the best option. As I have suggested, and will continue to, this book aims to be inclusive and comprehensive of families as much as possible, but nothing is better than getting to know the families yourself and making decisions together, based on scientific knowledge and evidence that health practitioners should bring and the expertise in themselves that families have.

The need to measure the impact of parental cancer on children was identified decades ago; however, there is still no 'gold standard' [73]. To date, there is no reliable data to show how infants and toddlers are affected by

Chapter Highlights

- Involving children and young people in cancer care is beneficial.
- Children and young people should be safe and comfortable, and their voices and opinions need to be considered.
- More family and child-friendly spaces should be encouraged.
- Families, children and healthcare practitioners should work as a 'team' and make decisions about the best support available to meet their needs.
- Emotional support and family support must be provided to support children, young people and families going through parental cancer.

parental cancer [73]. Except for a handful of countries, the majority lack accurate databases and a systematic way to register the number of cancer diagnosis and how many of these patients have children and young people.

5.2   Involving Children and Young People

Involving children in parental medical care has been identified as positive and beneficial for children and young people. It can have psychosocial benefits such as the capacity to normalize the experience of cancer for them and enabling them with a space to ask questions and learn about the illness [79]. Shared communication and decision-making can have a protective effect on the patient's psychological adjustment to cancer [47].

Healthcare practitioners have an important role in engaging children and young people, facilitating the creation of safe spaces for example where children and families can communicate and share together. Adolescents appreciated having access to the contact information of a health practitioner even though they may have never availed of it [9]. Weaver et al. [89] highlighted the need for oncology clinicians to support children by facilitating honest communication, maximising the child's support and facilitating open communication about cancer, and preparing the child for hospital visits and support through bereavement. Healthcare practitioners also need to promote a family-centred approach to talking to children about cancer [38]. Creating 'fit for purpose' spaces can reduce mistrust and tension between parents and children and can reduce psychological and social problems in the future [38]. Overall, adolescents wanted to be listened to personally, not advice from professionals [33]. I would add to that, particularly unwanted advice.

Involving children and young people implies a responsibility and commitment towards their care and well-being. Healthcare practitioners, if they decide to take on the role of supporting children and young people, have also a duty of care towards them. This can include providing emotional support. Healthcare practitioners can help young people understand the difference between anger towards the ill parent and anger at parental illness, as well as reducing adolescent guilt [11]. They can also support young people by reframing negative thoughts in more adaptive thoughts and adaptive ways whereby cancer is described as a serious illness, but it can be treated (if it can be), leading to hope and the capacity to understand and have more information about the illness [84]. Overall, adolescents described factual importance of being a 'normal' teenager and validating their feelings at the time of parental cancer [31]. Young people expressed appreciating the intervention of healthcare professionals in terms of validating their feelings of anger and guilt at the time of parental cancer [31].

Hospital visits and direct contact with medical staff can benefit children and young people, particularly those with a special interest in the medical side and treatment of cancer [45]. Maynard et al. [59] found that meeting the physician in charge of their parent's treatment was helpful as it was an opportunity for the child to ask questions but also 'humanised' the person who was undertaking their parent's care. Allowing children and young people to see the treatment facilities enabled young people to obtain more realistic information, rather than leaving it to their imagination only [59].

5.3 Child-Oriented Services

Literature generally agrees that health services are not usually child-friendly spaces, anywhere from infrastructure to actual willingness and skill, from professionals to engage with children and young people of adult patients. There is currently a need for targeted services for children and young people, but this is limited, for example, by the lack of clarity on the number of children affected by parental cancer; therefore, it is not possible to plan clinical practices with child-oriented services and provide recommendations for adult healthcare that is family friendly [118].

Research has found that children and young people that experience parental cancer have unmet needs that impact their experience of parental illness and their quality of life as well. Those children and young people with more unmet needs also experience higher levels of distress [119]. Therefore, child-oriented services are crucial to meet the needs of children and young people. Child-oriented services would benefit from multidisciplinary teams. Research has suggested that several factors act as mediating factors of child functioning when parents are diagnosed with cancer [49]. Some of these factors include appraisal of parental cancer, children's coping, psychosocial functioning, parenting quality, family functioning and family communication. Due to this combination of factors, families may benefit from a multidisciplinary support team including psychologists, social workers and oncology nurses to provide support and guidance to cancer patients [49]. These professionals, however, need additional training in child and family issues to be able to better support young families [49].

5.4 Selecting the 'Best' Supports

One of the challenges that healthcare practitioners have is selecting adequate support to match the needs of children, young person or families. In some cases, supports that are available are the only option for referral within the same health centres where a healthcare practitioner works; however, healthcare practitioners should be aware of support services available outside in the community or cancer support centres. Again, these decisions should be taken in conjunction with the families and given a choice, the best choices that they can select from.

Support groups for children and young people have been identified as a suitable way to engage children experiencing parental cancer. Support groups for children can provide them with an opportunity to express their worries and meet other children in similar situations, which can have a reassuring effect as they can bond as a community [38]. Parents that also provided feedback on these support groups felt that support groups reduced the burden on them by teaching children life skills and build the resilience of children which could help them to cope with parental cancer [38]. Some children, however, may also need and benefit from individual sessions if they are experiencing high levels of distress [38] at the time of parental cancer.

5.5 Information and Quality Sources

Cancer-related information was identified as the most prevalent unmet need in young people experiencing parental cancer [37]. Providing information to young people can reduce fear, uncertainty and misinformation associated with cancer [84]. Young people reported a strong need for information but did not know where to find answers for their cancer-related queries [10]. Research with children has emphasised that children would have liked to learn about their parent's illness as soon as possible after their parents were diagnosed, as well as having ongoing updates of their parents' condition [20]. Information needs varied; Kristjanson et al. [9] found that young people described their information needs as unique, depending on their personal and family characteristics, background knowledge about cancer, stage of their mothers' illness and their age.

The amount and type of information young people want was varied. Kristjanson et al. [9] identified that the most salient information that adolescents wanted to know was if their parent was going to survive. Information also included details about the seriousness of the illness, side effects, alternative therapies, medical facts, feelings and changes in their mothers and information about normal feelings. Jansson and Anderzen-Carlsson [8] found, for example, that young people were only interested in general facts about cancer and did not seek for any information beyond the one provided by their parents. Those who had searched only acknowledge that this information may be inaccurate [8]. Davey et al. [34] instead found that adolescents wanted to be informed and involved in their parent's treatment by attending appointments, searching for information in books, online and with physicians to fully understand the treatment.

Parents were identified as one of the most important sources of information; however, this also meant that they were 'guardians of information' and disclosed information according to their views on how much information and which information was appropriate [9]. McDonald et al. [25] found that families with high cohesion (togetherness, support) have higher levels of unmet needs regarding information, as it seems these families may not appreciate high levels of information needs and inhibit children and young people from asking. Some children, young people and families are interested in reading information and accessing information on their own in their own time; however, they may benefit from guidance regarding good and reliable sources [45]. Weeks et al. [120] carried out a scoping review to identify high-quality sources of information online for parents. This review identified seven sources that are still available (in 2021) and relevant and can be used to support parents and families when they experience a cancer diagnosis. Table 5.1 includes a description

Table 5.1 Sources of cancer information

Title	Author	Date	Description	Available at
Talking to children and teenagers when an adult has cancer	MacMillan Cancer Support (UK)	2016	Talking about cancer and treatments Children's reactions Coping Family life	https://cdn.macmillan.org.uk/dfsmedia/1a6f2353f7f4519b0cf14c45b2a629/803-source/talking-to-children-and-teenagers-when-an-adult-has-cancer-mac5766-e04-n
When a parent has cancer	University Health Network Canada	2017	Talking about cancer Coping Children's reaction Seeking help	www.uhn.ca/PatientsFamilies/Health_Information/Health_Topics/Documents/Tips_to_Build_Self_Regulation_Skills_Children_Parents_With_Cancer.pdf#search=parent%20cancer (Not exactly the same source)
Parenting at a challenging time	Massachusetts General Hospital Yale Cancer Centre	ND	Talking about cancer Developmental perspective Changes in family life Professional help Financial and legal issues Terminal cancer	www.yalecancercenter.org/patient/specialty/pact/ http://media-ns.mghcpd.org.s3.amazonaws.com/child-psychopharm-2016-child-psychopharm-sunday-rauch-parenting-at-a-challenging-time.pdf
Talking to Children about Cancer	Irish Cancer Society		Talking about cancer and treatments Children's reactions Family routines Terminal cancer	www.cancer.ie/cancer-information-and-support/cancer-support/coping-with-cancer/information-for-patients/talking-to-family-and-friends
Helping children when a family member has cancer: dealing with diagnosis	American Cancer Society	2012	Talking about cancer, diagnosis and treatment Children's reactions Coping	www.cancer.org/treatment/children-and-cancer/when-a-family-member-has-cancer.html

Table 5.1 (cont.)

Title	Author	Date	Description	Available at
Talking to kids about cancer	Cancer Council Australia	2015	Talking about cancer, diagnosis and treatment Family life Coping Terminal cancer	www.cancer.org.au/assets/pdf/talking-to-kids-about-cancer-a-guide-for-people-with-cancer-their-families-and-friends#:~:text=Practise%20your%20response%20to%20potential%20questions%20before%20talking%20to%20kids.and text=Explain%20that%20the%20cancer%20is%20not%20their%20fault%20and%20is%20not%20contagious.and text=Assure%20them%20they%20will%20always,t%20always%20do%20it%20yourself.and text=Stop%20and%20listen%20to%20your,know%20how%20they%20really%20feel.
Talking with your children about cancer	Breast Cancer Care (UK)	2014	Talking about cancer Children's reactions Seeking help After treatment	https://breastcancernow.org/sites/default/files/publications/pdf/bcc50_talking_to_your_children_2018_web.pdf

and summary of these seven sources as well as where they can be found online. These sources can be used by practitioners with confidence as they have been subject of a systematic evaluation.

> Age-appropriate rituals can enable children's symbolic meaning making as well as act as a reward for children's involvement and contribution in cancer care. For example, marking half of the treatment with half a cake [79].

5.6 Social Supports

Research has identified that social support is fundamental for children, young people and families coping with parental cancer, acting as a buffer the stress they experience at the time of illness [45] and helping families with emotional and concrete supports. Research has highlighted the role of family in supporting children and young people experiencing parental cancer. Adolescents experiencing parental cancer enjoyed spending time with parents and family but would benefit from comfort provided by other people [11]. Jorgensen et al. [121] found that social support was associated with adolescent well-being among adolescents experiencing parental cancer. Parents, siblings and other relatives have been identified as the main sources of support [34]. Even though family is the main source of social support identified, friends, peers, neighbours and extended family can also be significant sources of support at the time of parental cancer. Again, children and families can make decisions about the sources of support they would like to have, the frequency of contact and the type of support they feel comfortable obtaining from others.

Regarding peer supports, sharing the experience of parental cancer with friends was not common to all young people, some preferred not to divulge their parents' cancer at school to avoid unwanted attention, being teased or being asked on a regular basis about the situation [33, 34]. Healthcare practitioners can support young people by enabling and encouraging peer support. These support networks will enable communication with other young people who have gone through the same experience and encourage them to learn from each other [84]. Peers who have been through similar experiences can be very understanding towards young people and can reduce their feelings of loneliness [59].

School can also be an important source of social support, if children and young people are happy with it. Studies have identified that informing the school can be helpful, as teachers could be more understanding if they were aware of the situation the young person was going through, also reducing the pressure of school on young people [59]. Some young people appreciated support from school and being treated with a sense of normalcy [9]. Positive and compassionate staff members were also appreciated, but this excluded teachers 'overreacting', cuddling them or treating them differently because they had cancer [8]. Teachers can provide support to children and parents; however, these professionals also need to have the knowledge and skills to provide adequate support. Davey et al. [34] reported that one young person in their study described a bad experience with a healthcare practitioner who told her 'people often die of cancer' (p. 255).

Other families may benefit from other sources of support. Some studies mentioned community supports, including churches and neighbours as helpful towards their ill parent including providing food or flowers [9]. Adolescents, although described these supports as positive, they perceived that they experienced no support for themselves, but it was instead focused on their ill parent only [9].

5.7 Recommendations for Talking to Children and Young People

This book, so far, has provided recommendations from published scientific literature. One of the aspects they lack is more practical guidelines and pointers that can be found in manuals or booklets from 'grey' literature. This is due to the characteristic of scientific publications and their publication guidelines and format.

The following recommendations can be found online on websites from cancer support centres and organisations. In case you are interested in accessing these websites yourself they are included below. Additionally, Table 5.2 can be a useful resource that can be used when talking to parents about how to support children and cancer.

Table 5.2 Recommendations for talking to children and young people

Source	Website
Talking to children and teenagers when an adult has cancer. MacMillan Cancer Support.	www.macmillan.org.uk/cancer-information-and-support/diagnosis/talking-about-cancer/talking-to-children-and-teenagers
Talking with children about cancer.	www.cancer.net/coping-with-cancer/talking-with-family-and-friends/talking-about-cancer/talking-with-children-about-cancer
Talking to children about cancer.	www.cancer.ie/cancer-information-and-support/cancer-support/coping-with-cancer/information-for-patients/talking-to-family-and-friends
When your parent has cancer. A guide for teens.	www.cancer.gov/publications/patient-education/when-your-parent-has-cancer.pdf

5.8   Preparing Parents to Talk to Their Children and Young People

- **Timing**: A good time to talk is before obvious changes happen for example when the ill parent will lose their hair [122–124]. Children can cope with changes if they are told in advance.

- **Practice:** parents may benefit from writing down what they are going to say or try role play. The 'perfect' conversation does not exist and children may ask questions you were not expecting, hours or days later.

- **Company:** consider involving another person that you trust (and the children trust) to provide support. This can be a healthcare practitioner, a friend or a family member.

- **Frequency:** one conversation may not be enough. Brief and frequent conversations may be needed.

- **Open and honest:** parents should be open and honest about their diagnosis and their feelings. This will encourage trust and open communication from children. Parents should also use open questions: 'Tell me about….', 'How can we…?', 'What do you feel about…?'

- **Encourage questions:** children and young people need to know they can ask questions to their parents.

- **Visuals:** young children may benefit from visual aids such as books, drawings, dolls to explain cancer, where it is in the body, etc.

- **Location:** choose a comfortable environment at home. Spend time together doing familiar activities such as walking or playing. Avoid the child's room as this can be the child's 'safe place'. I have personally encouraged parents to plan a fun day out, allow some time for the child to listen and ask questions at home but then spend fun time together therefore the memories of such a hard disclosure will include happy family time memories also, if everyone is happy to do it. Some children might need more time to 'digest' the news or instead want to spend time on their own. Other sources [120] suggest telling children in a location away from home, which can become the place that you go back to when you want to talk about cancer. Avoid telling them at bedtime as they might not be able to sleep.

- **Others:** it might be useful to ask children, particularly young people, who else should know about cancer for example a teacher, a trainer, etc. Some young people may not want to tell their school or college to keep this place 'normal' for them. Others may instead want to tell the school to avail of support.

5.9   *Child-Friendly Cancer Glossary*

Table 5.3 includes a summary of common cancer terms in simple language, suitable for children [122–124].

Table 5.3 Child-friendly cancer terms

Term	Definition
Cancer	'There is something in my body called cancer. It is making me sick. The doctors are giving me medicine to try to make it go away'
Chemotherapy	Special medicine to get rid of the cancer.
	Drugs to cure or control cancer.
	Chemotherapy can make people feel sick, feel tired or lose their hair.
Tumour	Lump inside the body
Cells	Tiny building blocks in the body that group together (like building blocks) to build tissues and organs.
Radiotherapy	X-rays that can kill cancer cells.
	The skin can be red and sore.
	People can feel very tired
Surgery	Operation to remove the cancer or the part of the body where the cancer is.

5.10   Preparing Children and Young People for Hospital

Children and young people need to be prepared for hospital visits, in terms of how parents may look after treatments and surgery, for example if parents will have drips, tubes or any other machines [124]. The purpose of this is to help them feel better. Children and young people who want to look at scars can be allowed to do so; however, it might be better to do so when redness and swelling has decreased. Some may not want to see them at all and that should be respected also. Let children and young people know the different people that will be in the hospital to help you (doctors, nurses). Also, explain things to them like the call button, equipment, etc. Children and young people can bring books, game consoles, table, laptops, colour books or anything that might work for them. Families can have snacks and things they can do together such as games, word games, playing cards. If children or young people feel tired or overwhelmed, the adult who is with them can bring them home.

While you are in hospital try to keep contact with children, have a regular time to call them. Leave notes or small gifts for them to find while you are away. Send your children and young people a card or a letter. Stories or books can be read with young children over the phone or zoom.

Children and young people also need to know the side effects of treatments and understand that these effects may last even after treatments have finished. Having side effects is not a sign that the parent is getting sicker, not everyone gets the same side effects or in the same frequency. After treatment, you may feel tired and have side effects, children may expect their parent to get back to normal immediately after the treatment has been completed, however, they need to know that this may not happen.

Important information to share with children and young people [122–124]

- **Cancer:** explain the illness using the word cancer.
- **Health:** explain how your health will be affected.
- **Treatment:** explain treatment in simple and clear language.
- **Guilt:** children need to know they did not cause parental cancer and should not experience any guilt for it.
- **Cancer is not contagious:** you cannot catch it from one person to another. Closeness, affections (hugs and kisses) are still possible.
- **Care:** children need to be reassured that they will be taken care of (preferably with information of by who and that they know and get along with this person).
- **Communication:** reassure children and young people that they can ask questions and express how they feel, they will be listened to.
- **Speed:** give information to children slowly, repeat the information so the message is clear until the children are comfortable with it.
- **Truth:** avoid too many details about cancer, finances, or test results but everything you say should be the truth, do not make promises that you cannot keep.
- **Listen:** encourage children to talk, express their thoughts and emotions (if they want to).
- **Share:** express your feelings as well as cancer information.
- **Reassure:** let the children know that they are still loved and cared for.

5.11   The Developmental Approach

Table 5.4 summarises different sources regarding recommendations on how to speak to children about cancer, reaction and ways to support them by age group [122–124].

5.12   Child-Friendly Bibliography[1]

This is a compilation of different sources that provided information about children's books about cancer (Table 5.5). These books can support parents as well as healthcare practitioners when explaining cancer to children and young people. Visual aids such as this can help children understand cancer and its treatment as well as associated emotions and possible side effects. I have not personally used all of these books. I have marked those that I have used before.

---

[1]   www.huffpost.com/entry/childrens-books-about-cancer_l_5e32f5efc5b611ac94d0e347
   www.yalecancercenter.org/patient/specialty/pact/booklist/
   https://breastcancernow.org/about-us/news-personal-stories/tools-talking-children-about-cancer
   https://childrenslitlove.com/2020/02/05/childrens-books-about-cancer/

Table 5.4 Recommendations to talk by age group

Age group	Communication	Reaction	How to support them
Babies and toddlers	Cannot understand cancer.	Sensitive on changes in the routine and their carer.	Keep environments familiar and consistent.
	Parents should tell them about upcoming events in simple, clear and reassuring language.	Might be scared that medical staff will separate them from their parents and take medical tests.	Choose someone to care for the child who is familiar to them.
	Let children for how long you will be away/ in hospital (if you know for sure)		Keep routines familiar.
	'Mammy is sick'		Give children plenty of love and attention.
	'Daddy needs to go to the hospital'		
Children 3 to 5	Children can understand cancer in simple terms.	Children can perceive tension and physical emotional changes in adults.	Reassure that cancer is not their fault.
	Explain that treatment is used to make them feel better.	They react to changes in routine and separations so they might become 'clingy' and scared of parental separation.	Use a doll, teddy bear or doll to explain places where the cancer is located, treatments, etc.
	Explain that doctors can make treatments less painful.	They think hopes and wishes will cure their parent.	Keep everyday routines, limits and boundaries.
		They can experience guilt and regressive behaviours (thumb-sucking, bed-wetting, tantrums), become quiet and have bad dreams.	Ask someone they know and trust to mind them.

Children 6 to 12	Children can understand a more detailed explanation of cancer. Can understand that medicine and treatments will make the parent feel better. Be honest about pain and treatment side effects. Children can listen to cancer information from other sources such as TV, Internet, peers, etc. Encourage shared conversations to avoid worry.	Children can understand more explanations about cancer and its effects. Fear can include death or 'catching' cancer. They will set high standards to be 'good'. Changes are expected in behaviour, concentration, schoolwork, friendships, eating habits, sleeping patterns, etc.	Cancer books can be read together. Keep their activities, school and friendships going. Give them small tasks they can use to help. Allow them to enjoy themselves and have fun.
Teenagers	Can understand a complex explanation of cancer. Might be interested in more details about diagnosis and treatment. Listen to cancer messages from different sources and encourage discussions.	Teenagers understand cancer but may struggle to talk about it and express their feelings.	Provide sources of information. Knowledge can stop young people from imagining that the reality is worse. Include them, invite them to ask questions and express feelings. Normalise young people's feelings. Encourage time to spend time on their own. Keep rules and limits. Allow them to be involved in more household activities as a sign that they are needed and trusted but show appreciation for the help.
Children with disabilities and/or special needs	Children may struggle to understand changes due to illness.	Children can find change difficult	Explain new things in a way that has worked before. Need to stick to routines. Repeat illness explanations as many times as needed, use the same simple words.

Table 5.5 Cancer books for children

Author	Title	Description
Abigail Ackerman	Our mum has cancer	Abigail and Adrienne tell their experience of maternal cancer over a year (4–8 years).
Alex, Emily and Anna Rose Silver	Our dad is getting better.	Children's experience on how their father was recovering from cancer treatment.
Alex Silver	Our mum is getting better.	This book addresses survivorship to help families to move on after treatment ends (4–8 years).
American Cancer Society	Because …Someone I love has cancer	This is an activity book for children that uses artwork to let children express when a loved one has cancer (6–12 years).
Amy Rovere	And still they bloom.	This is a story book about the story of two children who grieve the loss of their mother in different ways.
Anita Howell	B is for breast cancer	Lucy and Jack describe their experience of maternal breast cancer. The book includes medical treatments suitable for young children.
Ann Speltz	The year my mother was bald.	This is a book for older children to understand cancer from a scientific standpoint.
Carol Carrick	Upside-down cake.	This book is from the perspective of a 9-year-old boy whose father had terminal cancer.
Carol Weston	Melanie Martin goes Dutch.	In this book Melanie Martin goes on a summer vacation with her family and friend whose mother has breast cancer.
Carrie Martin	The rainbow feelings of cancer.	The book contains the writing and drawings of a young girl and her experience of maternal cancer (9–12 years).
Christine Clifford	Our family has cancer too!	This is a cartoon book which encourages conversation between parents and children (9–12 years).
Debbie Watters	Where's Mom's Hair	This book is narrated by a son who explains cancer treatment and recovery (4–8 years).
Eileen Sutherland	Mom and the polka-dot booboo: A gentle story explaining breast cancer to a young child.	A story to explain breast cancer to young children (4–8 years).
Elizabeth Winthrop	Promises	In this book a girl describes her day-to-day life as her mother goes through cancer treatment (4–8 years).
*Ellen McVicker	Butterfly kisses and wishes on wings.	Provides a child-friendly explanation on cancer. It addresses common questions that children may have.

Eva Grayzel	You are not alone: Families touched by cancer	Children around the world share their experiences of having a family member with cancer (9–12 years).
Gillian Forrest	Mummy's Lump	This is a book for families that want to talk to their young children about breast cancer.
Genevieve Castree	A Bubble	This book is the personal experience of a mother diagnosed with cancer and her young daughter.
Helen Welsh	The perfect shelter	This book is about cancer, family relationships, love and support for the ill family member.
Janna Matthies	The goodbye cancer garden.	In this book a family plants a garden as their mother experiences cancer treatment and recovery (4–8 years).
Jessica Reid Sliwerski	Cancer hates kisses.	Written by a breast cancer survivor. This book is told from the perspective of a child whose mother is experiencing cancer.
Julie Aigner Clark	You are the best medicine.	This book is focused on how children cared for their ill mother and how mothers care for and nurture children over their life course.
Katherine Hannigan	Ida B	This a book about a young girl's struggles following maternal cancer diagnosis (9+ years).
Kelly A. Tinkham	Hair for mama.	This book is the view of an 8-year-old boy whose mother had cancer.
Laura Numeroof and Wendy Harpham	The hope tree: Kids talk about breast cancer	The book is about a fictional support group for animals whose mother have cancer (experiences, worries and coping)
*Marge Eaton Heegaard	When someone has a very serious illness: children can learn to cope with loss and change.	This book supports children with thoughts and feelings that arise when a family member is experiencing serious illness.
National Cancer Institute	When your parent has cancer	A guide for young people who have a parent with cancer.
Patricia Polacco	The Lemonade Club	The book is based on a true story of a girl who helped a friend and her teacher through cancer.
Ruth Pennebaker	Both sides now.	A 15-year-old girl's life writes about her experience of maternal cancer.
Sara Olsher	Cancer Party! Explain cancer, chemo, and radiation to kids in a totally non-scary way.	This book is the conversation of a mother explaining a cancer diagnosis to her 6-year-old daughter.

Table 5.5 (cont.)

Author	Title	Description
Shenin Sachedina	Metu and Lee learn about breast cancer	The book helps understand cancer and how it affects women (5+ years)
Sue Glader	Nowhere Hair	This book helps children understand cancer and treatment, fear and sadness with humour and rhyme (4–8 years).
Vanessa Bayer	How do you care for a very sick bear?	Written by a teenage leukaemia survivor to explain how children can support others through cancer treatment.

* These are books I have used in therapy myself

5.13 Implications for Practice

- Receiving information from healthcare staff has been described as beneficial for children and young people, particularly associated with feelings of trust that the sick parent is properly taken care of as well as it increases the ability to understand the diagnosis more than if information was received from their parents only [125].

- Open and instructive communication with healthcare practitioners enables family members to be more involved, ask questions about the diagnosis, prognosis and treatment [125].

- Adolescents would benefit from open communication, being available and feeling that they are being taken seriously. This will give them the confidence to speak and acquire the knowledge they want through the different stages of parental cancer [125].

- Healthcare practitioners can provide opportunities for young people to interpret and validate new information [10].

- Professionals should evaluate needs individually, rather than assuming that the information needs of all children, adolescents and families are equal [9].

Card Activity [84]

In this activity, questions are printed on small cards and these cards are scattered in the centre of the room for participants to select them one at a time, read the card out loud and answer in the way they wish to.

- Why do good people get cancer?
- How does it feel to have a family member with cancer?
- Is it okay to feel sad, angry, lonely if someone in your family has cancer?

Chapter 6

Evidence-Based Cancer Interventions

6.1 Introduction

This book, so far, has explored and described in depth the issues, experiences and emotions that a cancer diagnosis brings to children, adolescents and families. As a health practitioner I would like to know how to best support children and families in these circumstances. As you read through the chapter, please be aware that this is a review of the current knowledge regarding interventions that have been published. Therefore, it does not include all the possible interventions available, only those published in the academic or grey research available at the time of literature search for this book. This, however, is still an opportunity to critically evaluate the current knowledge available. This means that this is an opportunity to learn from the successes but also the limitations of colleagues around the world regarding interventions.

This also means that if you have your own intervention and it is successful, you can share it. Interventions of course need to be systematically evaluated to be accepted and evidence based but if you know this can help children and families, it is important to 'spread the voice', learn from each other and continually improve practice and inform policy. This is an area where knowledge is currently scarce, even more in some parts of the world. The paradox is that cancer is a critical issue that affects children and families all over the world.

Chapter Highlights

- Interventions to support children and families exist but need to be evaluated with more rigorous methodologies to ensure their effectiveness.
- Lack of agreement of interventions outcomes makes comparisons between interventions impossible.
- Most effective interventions include core components but have the flexibility to adapt to the changing needs of children and families.
- Core components of interventions include provision of information, improving communication, expressing emotional skills, increasing social support and identifying and enhancing coping strategies.

Cancer affects thousands of children, adolescents and families worldwide every year. The World Health Organisation [126] estimated that cancer is responsible for over ten million deaths in 2020. The National Cancer Institute in the United States [127] calculated that there were 18.1 million new cases of cancer diagnosed in the world, and estimated that by 2040, the number of new cases will rise to 29.5 million. There are no reliable statistics of how many of these diagnoses correspond to parents of children and young people, but it is highly likely that many of these people diagnosed will have families that will be affected by a cancer diagnosis.

Research has identified that children and young people affected by cancer may not have their needs met when a parent or carer is diagnosed with cancer. Specifically, they may have unmet needs regarding how to deal with feelings, high levels of distress and family relationships [37]. This suggests the need for counselling and psychological interventions for young people experiencing parental cancer [37, 128]. And this also justifies the need for effective ways to meet the needs of children and families through programmes or interventions, but not any of them, good ones, effective ones. The obvious response to this would be to deliver programmes or interventions that can respond to those needs, however, this is not currently without its challenges.

Ohan et al. [129] adapted the six key needs of children of parents with cancer to psychosocial interventions. These key needs that they identified were:

1. Give children age-appropriate information about parental cancer.
2. Support children in communication with their parents and family.
3. Peer support can be used to normalise and reduce feelings of isolation.
4. Facilitate children with a safe space to express their feelings.
5. Tailor individual coping and support for children in distress.
6. Children who experience bereavement may need specialised supports and connections.

Ohan et al. [129] found that at the time, not a single intervention approached each of the six components. The most common component approached was family communication and the least was bereavement support. The programmes that included the most components were Children of Somatically Ill Parents (COSIP) [130], Wonders and Worries [128], Children's Lives Include Moments of Bravery (CLIMB) (Japanese version) [131] and FOCUS [132]. These interventions are described in more detail in this chapter.

One of the challenges that currently exist specifically regarding the selection and appropriateness of interventions is the lack of empirical research on interventions and insufficient methodological rigour which has been used to evaluate some of them. This means that there is a lack of guidance in selecting interventions [129] and I would add, good and evidence-based interventions, that ideally would make a health practitioner feel completely confident to use them with the families they are working with.

Existing interventions are limited in terms of their evidence and quality. Alexander et al. [81] carried out a systematic review of current interventions available to support children living with a parent with cancer and concluded that studies were underpowered, lacked standardisation, randomisation and controls. These limitations were also identified by other research studies [133]. There is a large proportion of qualitative evaluations for interventions and heterogeneity in outcome measures across studies [130], which means the impact of interventions cannot be fairly compared in terms of outcomes and impact on families. There is a need for more rigorous evaluation methodologies that can identify evidence-based interventions, including, for example pre- and post-evaluations of child and family functioning [134, 135]. Research is needed to find short and sensitive instruments to measure the effectiveness of an intervention [136].

Research on family interventions is also limited by the fact that existent research is focused on the dominant culture family structures and less is known about the broader spectrum of families, culture values and practices [137]. Interventions included in this chapter are focused on interventions mainly carried out in Europe and the United States. Less is known about other regions of the world. This does not mean that culturally sensitive interventions do not exist, it means they might need more availability to the public. Another challenge of interventions is regarding the content and design, some interventions lack an underpinning theory to inform the development and implementation [81] of interventions. Family interventions may not fit the broader theoretical framework underpinning research studies [132] in which they have been included. Interventions that have an underpinning theoretical framework are deemed as more trustworthy and robust and it is therefore one criterion which can be used to evaluate the quality of interventions.

Dosage of interventions is also unclear, therefore more research is needed to consider the dose of interventions that are required to achieve benefits and positive outcomes, as well as under which conditions, to ensure the desired effect of the interventions is achieved [136]. It is also important to understand if there is a possibility to extend the duration of the effect of an intervention and how best to achieve these lasting effects [136]. More research is needed to determine if booster sessions are required, and the timeframe needed for these to be effective. Northouse et al. [132] described that some families may need more sessions if the cancer progressed and some other families might need very specific interventions, shorter and more limited in time.

Another challenge is reality. Cancer can be an 'unpredictable' illness and depending on the prognosis, impact of treatments, family circumstances and needs may change very rapidly. Interventions should be based on the needs of children and young people; the challenge however is that these needs may change over time and support programmes should be adapted and adaptable to these changing needs [132]. This may not be practical or possible in the short term due to the time and resources needed to properly evaluate an intervention.

This means that healthcare practitioners have evidence to trust that the intervention creates benefits and positive outcomes and protects families and children from adversity or negative outcomes, in an already challenging and vulnerable circumstance. Other issues identified are the need for transparency with regard to staff skills and whether staff or volunteers oversaw delivery of interventions. This may impact the delivery and therefore the effectiveness of interventions [87].

In the following sections, this chapter will focus on describing existing interventions for children and families that have been evaluated (to different degrees of rigour). It will critically describe the methods of delivery, activities and dynamics, including practical activities. Finally, the chapter intends to identify common components and parameters that those effective interventions have included as suggested pillars of interventions to meet the needs of children and families who experience parental cancer.

6.2   Interventions for Children and Families

Interventions to support children, young people and families are crucial at a stressful and challenging time such as parental cancer. Families of cancer patients can provide substantial amounts of unpaid care for patients and can be affected by the social, emotional, physical and spiritual well-being of families [136]. Therefore, family interventions can be an alternative to support families experiencing parental cancer. All family members, including children and the healthy parent, should be included in psychosocial interventions [85, 138].

Several research studies have advocated for the need of having family-centred interventions with families experiencing cancer [17]. Some interventions were targeted at parents specifically. Stafford et al. [139], for example, designed and evaluated a psycho-educational intervention specifically targeted at improving parental efficacy and reducing parental stress targeted at parents with children between 3 and 12 years of age. Interventions should empower parents to feel that they are able to talk with their children and support them [17]. Parents of adolescents also need to feel secure in supporting young people [8]. The need to include family in interventions was also confirmed by adolescents themselves. Davey et al. [33] identified that adolescents wanted to involve their parents to increase group attendance. Several studies have provided insights into the components needed for family interventions.

A variety of interventions were analysed and their components included the following [20, 94, 140, 141]:

1. Psychoeducation: Additional information about cancer, treatments and clarifying misconceptions. Cancer treatment centre tours.

2. Supportive counselling.

3. Coping skills (coping with stress).

4. Communication enhancement.

5. Affective involvement.

6. Family functioning.
7. Improve child and parental adjustment.
8. Family relationships and cohesion.
9. Reduce isolation.
10. Normalise and cope with emotions.
11. Hope for the future.

Northouse [136] identified some of the elements that should be included in family interventions for families experiencing cancer:

1. Interventions should be jointly considered between patients and caregivers. This enables a mutual understanding of needs and perceptions that enables more effective teamwork.

2. Interventions need to deliver core content, but content should also be tailored to the needs of each family.

3. Support families in identifying sources of support available to them to increase their social networks such as friends and neighbours.

4. Encourage active coping strategies in families, for example problem solving and decision-making.

5. Determine the meaning of the illness for families to identify the unexpected benefits that may be associated with cancer.

6. Provide practical information on how to manage symptoms including fatigue, pain, sleep disturbances and hormonal changes.

7. Families may need help identifying information from healthcare providers and reliable sources of information online.

8. Families may need support in dealing with multiple demands and may need permission to limit work and other family and personal responsibilities.

Eilis et al. [134] carried out a systematic review exploring the psychosocial needs and existing interventions for children facing parental cancer. This study identified five critical aspects that need to be included in an intervention with children:

1. Age-appropriate information about parental cancer to avoid misconceptions about cancer which may be more frightening than the reality of their parent's illness.

2. Support children to communicate with parents, family members and health professionals.

3. Provide a safe environment where children can share their emotions and normalise their experiences with peers.

4. Specialised support for bereavement and coping with parental death.

5. Interventions should be sensitive to gender and racial differences [33]. Groups would also benefit from facilitators from different genders and racially matched with families [33].

Oja et al. [142] also supported the need to increase knowledge and understanding in children as this dispels misconceptions and enables more understanding about illness in the family. Open communication enables children and young people to speak out and gives them a sense of relief as they have a safe place to speak. Interventions also encouraged agency to identify opportunities to provide small practical tasks to support families and the need to find opportunities for 'escapism', having fun and balancing their lives with parental needs [142].

Northouse et al. [132] designed and evaluated the FOCUS programme. This programme consists of five components and has been evaluated with women experiencing recurrent breast cancer and their families. These components are described in Table 6.1.

Wonders and Worries was designed and evaluated in the United States for children dealing with parental cancer [128]. According to the authors, one of the strengths of this intervention is that it has an underpinning theoretical model and is curriculum based. The themes included in the curriculum are individualised to the needs of each family, the developmental stage of the child and children's activity choices such as games or artistic activities. The tailoring of the intervention enabled the inclusion of families from a variety of settings and different illness stages. This is relevant because, for example regarding information, it was found that information about cancer may be more helpful for families with a newly diagnosed parent, families who have a diagnosis for longer time may need a different type of content [94].

The impact of the evaluation was measured in a period of five years [128]. The intervention consists of six sessions that provide age-appropriate illness information which can support children and adolescents to cope with stress and fear related to parental cancer. This intervention promoted positive adaptation for children and families including improved communication skills, less anxiety, more security at home and improved educational outcomes [128]. The sessions of the Wonders and Worries programme are summarised in Table 6.2.

Nelson [144] designed a parallel group programme which is based on the principle that children's experience of parental cancer is dependent on family communication and family functioning. This group was targeted at families of patients parenting children between 5 and 18 years of age; however, they were divided into age-specific groups. To suit families, the group was also carried out in the evenings (6–8 pm) and food was provided. The group is run by oncology staff and trained volunteers, and past participants can become mentors to new families as well.

Referred families are assessed regarding communication patterns within the family, children's special needs and suitability for the group. Before joining families are informed of the group format and that fact that deaths are 'honoured' in the group. Nelson [143], however, included a word of caution;

Table 6.1 Components of the FOCUS programme

	Components	Subcomponents
F	Family involvement	**Promote open communication:** families varied in the degree that they communicated openly about cancer.
		Encourage mutual support and teamwork: importance of mutual support was discussed.
		Identify family strength: family strengths were identified and encouraged.
		Helping children in the family: families struggled to communicate with their children. Discussions about cancer provided opportunities to talk about cancer within families.
O	Optimistic attitude	**Practice optimistic thinking:** families struggled to be optimistic particularly when facing recurrence.
		Share feelings and negative thoughts: share fears about recurrence that undermine their capacity to feel optimistic.
		Maintain hope: families were encouraged to focus on positive aspects of their experiences and to reframe negative events when possible.
		Staying hopeful in the face of death: patients and families were given permission to maintain hope despite the situation they were experiencing.
C	Coping effectiveness	**Dealing with overwhelming stress:** recurrence was challenging and overwhelming for families.
		Encourage healthy coping and lifestyle behaviours: families shared what they did to cope with stress. Coping strategies and healthy lifestyles were discussed with all patients and families.
		Helping caregivers manage the demands of the illness: caregivers were often overwhelmed and distressed due to their roles and changes in their lives.
U	Uncertainty reduction	**Obtaining information:** families were provided with facts about cancer, recurrence and treatments.
		Learning to be assertive: when families expressed that their questions were not answered adequately, they were encouraged to be assertive and request healthcare providers for more information.
		Learning to live with uncertainty: uncertainty is associated with fear that the treatment will not work, and the cancer would be terminal. The intervention was not intended to eliminate uncertainty but to support families in managing it.
S	Symptom management	**Assessing symptoms:** families described the physical and emotional symptoms they were experiencing (pain, fatigue, nausea, anorexia, etc.).
		Teaching self-care strategies: facilitators (nurses) provided families with pre-printed symptom management cards.

Table 6.2 Components of the Wonders and Worries programme

Session		Description
1	Getting to know each other	Build rapport between participants and facilitators to facilitate a sense of safety to discuss sensitive topics.
2	Cancer education	Developmentally tailored education about cancer, treatment and side effects.
3	Cancer treatment centre tour	Tour of the cancer centre and equipment as well as education about the treatment plan.
4	Feelings	Support to identify and label feelings that the family is experiencing related to the illness.
5	Stress and coping	Define stress and identify ways of coping that children and young people use to deal with the stress. Provide alternative ideas such as sports, play with pets, journaling and arts.
6	Hopes for the future/ closure	Focus on hope for the future, positive things may evolve from difficult circumstances, identify potential positive things that have happened since the diagnosis.

multiple deaths in the group can have a negative emotional impact on the group, particularly those participants who are dealing with their own experience of death in the family.

Table 6.3 describes some of the activities used in the intervention for specific age groups.

Overall, interventions targeted at supporting children and young people should be developmentally appropriate. Interventions should include children but also encourage their meaningful participation [81]. Research has found that the quality and quantity of information provided to children relates to the way they coped, both during the illness and with bereavement [4]. Professionals have a role in ensuring that children are involved in discussions and information sharing in the way and extent chosen by them [94]. There is a particular lack of interventions for very young children between 0 and 5 years of age, therefore there is also a limited understanding of how best to support very young children [69].

Content should be available for families to decide which content they want to access in a way that will be useful to them [94]. Interventions should also be adapted to specific settings (inpatient/outpatient care) as well as consider the situation of families, for example the physical ability of an ill parent [141].

Table 6.3 Intervention activities per age group

Age group	Activities
Children group (5–12 years)	1. Art and play are used to enhance communication and participation. 2. Opening Circle: 'talking stick' is used to share information about who is sick. Children ask a fun question to each other. 'Popcorn-sharing' is used to talk about a specific theme. Relaxation and meditation techniques are taught. 3. Play: high and low energy areas are used to work through strong emotions. It includes board games, medical play area, soft building block, dollhouse, Lego, dodgeball, Twister, bowling. 4. Closing Circle: share the art activity. Participants make a wish for the month (out loud or quietly) by placing a ceramic heart in a bowl.
Teen group (13–18 years)	1. Group structure is flexible as group attendance fluctuates. 2. Music is played in the background; teenagers are asked to bring music to share.
Parent group	1. Support education on how to parent through cancer is provided. 2. Peer support is encouraged.
Death ceremony	1. When somebody dies, hearts are passed around in each group to honour the person.
Family group	2. This is a closing ritual where all family members are brought together, children share their art activity. 3. All participants hold hands and pass around a hand squeeze.

6.3 Delivery

Interventions were delivered online as well as face to face. Both have their own advantages and limitations that will be described below.

6.3.1 Online

Online interventions are especially useful for families that cannot access face to face services due to their location [87]. Morris [87] has described that the complexity of interventions has grown enabling the delivery of more targeted supports such as social supports, emotional supports, online parenting and family interventions. Another advantage of online interventions is that they can adapt more easily to family schedules and restrictions. According to Bingisser et al. [141], it is unlikely to be able to deliver 20 hours of face-to-face counselling to a family within four months of a cancer diagnosis. Online interventions can be accessed irrespective of day, time and place. Families can also select the content that is relevant to them and choose how much time they spend online. Online interventions, however, may not be suitable for everyone. Jansson and Anderzen-Carlsson [8] found that adolescents had concerns about finding peers online including privacy and anonymity.

6.3.2 Combined

Stafford et al. [139] considered (even before the COVID-19 pandemic) that there is a desire in healthcare organisations to deliver interventions with a combination of technological and face to face methodologies. Clinical contact by phone can be used with individual patients and/or their families facilitating tailoring to individual characteristics and needs [139]. Online and audio-visual resources are described as relatively inexpensive and highly accessible media to share and access information [139].

6.3.3 Face to face

Semple and McMaughan [20] carried out an intervention face to face with children as this enabled the provision of peer support that online programs cannot provide. The importance of this was to provide a relaxed and fun environment where children who had a shared experience could normalise their experience and reduce their feelings of isolation [20]. O'Neill et al. [16] evaluating the CLIMB programme, stated that meeting other children in a similar situation had a calming effect and enabled the children to bond as a community. This was also the case for CLIMB in Japan, where children and families expressed being able to share their feelings as a family but also valued the opportunity to share with others who were experienced similar situations [145].

Davey et al. [33] found that adolescents thought having a group of other young people close to the diagnosis, would have been helpful. Some, however, explained that they would have liked to attend a same-sex group, as male adolescents may not open as much with females in the group [33]. On the contrary, Ohan et al. [129] facilitated peer support by creating an online group for adolescents over 12 years. These enabled adolescents affected by parental cancer to interact with each other. Therefore, peer support can also be created and provided online.

6.4 Activities and Materials

This section includes, in more detail, some of the activities described and included in intervention articles. These activities include art, music, mindfulness, yoga, poetry, relaxation, Tai Chi, etc.

- Art is a medium of personal expression which has shown to reduce pain, reduce stress, increase awareness, improve wellness and improve the experience for cancer survivors [137]. These methods can also be used as means of expression for family members who may struggle to verbally express their emotions.

- Music has proven to be useful to decrease anxiety, depression, mood disturbances and pain related to cancer, as well as evoke strong emotions, validate feelings of power and hope, identified also in studies with cancer patients and families [137].

- Poetry is a form of creative and written expression which contributes to physical and emotional recovery, as well as exploring, reframing experiences deeply [137].

- Tai Chi has been demonstrated to be useful in reducing anxiety and depression, increasing relaxation, improving sleeping patterns and providing social support for families of breast cancer survivors [137]. Additionally, movements, relaxation and meditation components of Tai Chi increase balance, strength and well-being [137].

- Yoga has been used in cancer patients and survivors, proving to be capable of improving mental health and physical well-being as well as increase self-awareness [137].

- Mindfulness based stress reductions techniques have shown to improve mood, emotional disability, stress, poor concentration and strained family relationships [137].

- Relaxation exercises [94].

- Handicrafts [94].

- Stories and story books which were particularly appreciated by young children [92].

- Diaries (to write and draw) and or workbooks can work for children as a 'life recall' where they can continue the connection with the parent who has died [94, 129].

- Drawing and writing are used with small children as these have been described as methodologically appropriate to explore their understanding and experiences of illness [20].

- Audio-visual resources (DVD) [139].

- Online information, pamphlets and videos [129].

- Question List: consists of a set of predetermined questions that patients may wish to ask their health professionals. These are meant to empower patients to ask questions they wouldn't have asked otherwise [139].

- A phone call with a clinical psychologist [139].

6.5 Outcomes

This section includes a summary of the kinds of outcomes that have been measured in evaluations. One important aspect to take into consideration is that the outcomes measured should be justified based on the current knowledge about the issues and difficulties that families experiencing parental cancer have. Some of these outcomes are negative, suggesting that families only experience negative outcomes. This is not true, as previous chapters have described. Instead, practitioners should be encouraged to identify positive outcomes as well as negative ones. Not including measures to capture all types of outcomes means a lost opportunity to understand the experience of cancer for families in a more comprehensive way. These outcomes include:

- Depression. Interventions have been effective to reduce levels of depression [81, 135, 145].
- Reduced anxiety [135, 145].
- Post-traumatic stress disorder [81].
- Emotional regulation [81].
- Dealing with emotions [94].
- Enhanced coping strategies [94, 141].
- Improved sleep [140].
- Improved sense of security [140].

Careful consideration should be put into the design and evaluation on interventions, as this will enable the anticipation of potential barriers [141]. A cancer diagnosis can affect an entire family, and families with complex schedules may have difficulties to engage and adhere to interventions [94].

O'Neill et al. [17] emphasise the need for appropriate screening processes to support parents and children, obtain background information and determine if interventions in terms of content and modality of delivery are appropriate for the needs of a child and their family or not. Appropriate follow-ups need to be in place, for example an individual follow-up session with parents and children to reinforce the skills and learning acquired in the intervention to empower families to continue to use the tools and schools learnt in the programme [17]. Some children may also require follow-up support if they are continuing to experience significant levels of distress post-intervention [17].

6.6 Interventions for Practitioners

Interventions for healthcare professionals have been designed and evaluated as well. These interventions have the objective of empowering end educating practitioners on how best to work with children, young people and families.

Semple [5] delivered an online intervention which included the following content:

1. Provide a platform for practitioners to reflect on their beliefs about communication with families.
2. Integrate e-learning into routine clinical practice to facilitate learning and transmission of skills and knowledge.

3. Learn about behaviour change techniques that can be applied in practice.

4. Learn skills to empower parents to support and communicate with children and support parents.

5. Provide skills on age-appropriate language to communicate with children about cancer.

Moore et al. [146] systematically evaluated communication skills training for healthcare practitioners. Effective communication and support from healthcare practitioners can contribute to reduce stress in patients and their families and it is therefore a crucial skill that can be learnt and improved on. Some studies have questioned the current knowledge that exists about essential skills and have described the evidence as weak [147, 148]. This area, therefore, would benefit from further exploration.

The skills and recommendations for effective communication with people with cancer are [146]:

1. Use information gathering skills: open questions, facilitation, clarifying and summarising.

2. Discover the patient's perspective: elicit concerns, checking understanding, negotiate procedures and future arrangements.

3. Incorporate a psychosocial assessment.

4. Supportive relationships skills: showing empathy towards patients, respond to emotions and offer support.

5. Provide facts only.

The potential pitfalls may include [146]:

1. Leading questions.

2. Focus on the physical aspects, excluding the psychological issues.

3. Providing premature reassurance.

Several media have been used to deliver interventions for practitioners including videos, case studies and problem-solving exercises.

- Videos. Semple [5] used a series of videos as part of delivery. These videos included a variety of topics: (1) dialogue between a parent and a healthcare practitioner on how to talk to children about cancer. (2) Manage potential resistance to share by parents. (3) Reflection on sharing communication with children. Videos included real parents and children [149].

- Case discussions.

- Problem-solving exercises.

- Role-play is based on clinical examples [149].

- Individual sessions [145].

- Couple sessions [145].

- Group sessions [145].
- Art therapy [145].
- Music therapy [145].
- Bibliotherapy: books can provide help through alternative perspectives of how other people have coped with a similar situation [84].
- Relaxation and visualisation can facilitate the release of tension and anxiety [84].

Visualisation Exercise [84]

a) Visualise the negative emotional state in a metaphorical way (e.g. a blanket covering a body).

b) Transform the image in the mind (e.g. shedding sadness by shedding the blanket).

c) Create a new image accompanied by a more neutral feeling to replace the negative one (e.g. blanket is replaced by a puffy cloud floating in the sky).

d) Learn how to use the sadness in a more adaptive way.

6.7 School-Based Interventions

Research has suggested that teachers can have a crucial role in supporting children and young people, particularly in recognising and responding to their levels of distress [150]. Young people found comforting that teachers were aware of parental cancer as this enabled them to express feelings honestly and have permissions to miss school if they attended appointments with their ill parent [8]. Therefore, the more knowledgeable the school staff have about cancer, the better it will enable them to be more prepared to respond sensitively to the children and families facing parental cancer as well as provide leadership at a community level [150]. Teachers as community practitioners may have the advantage of having a professional relationship with a family prior to the diagnosis. This means that they may also have a deeper and more thorough understanding of family communication styles and functioning, reducing their fear [4].

Fasciano et al. [150] designed and evaluated the programme called 'When a Parent Has Cancer: Strengthening the School's Response'. This programme targeted schoolteachers specifically. School-based interventions included the following components:

- Provide facts about cancer and its treatment.
- Inform teachers about services available in the community where they could refer families who need help.

- Develop an age appropriate understanding of the illness in children .
- Discuss parental emotional experiences of cancer.
- Consider the role of school professionals in supporting children and families.

How to Make Love Tokens [63]

To make my love tokens, I got some card and cut out some heart shapes and decorated them with different words. You could write a hug token, a cuddle token, a treat token, a time token, a giggle token and a foot rub token. You might be able to come up with some even better ones!

When you have finished, place the love tokens in a box, bag or jar. You can make up your own rules about how you use tokens. It could be that you decide everyone gets to choose a token once a day – in the morning or when you come home from school or maybe at the dinner table. You can trade in your love token for whatever it says on the front. I love our token times as we really connect as a family.

6.8 Implications for Practice

In an 'ideal' world as a health practitioner, I would like to be able to tailor all interventions to the specific needs of children and families. I am aware that tailoring interventions may not always be possible due to limited time and budgets in health centres as well as other issues such as understaffing and high demand of services. What I am proposing, based in the evidence, is to include thematic components, flexible enough to be selected based on needs and the length of support families are willing to accept and commit to. Interventions, to be effective, need to be culturally and contextually sensitive. Some interventions were also tailored to different illness stages.

The common contents across interventions are:

1. Provide age-appropriate information about cancer, treatment and side effects.
2. Improve communication between parents, children and families, as well as healthcare practitioners.
3. Facilitate expression of emotions in a safe environment.
4. Increase social support for families.
5. Identify and enhance coping strategies.

In conclusion, the best interventions will not work if families, but mostly children and young people feel obliged to attend. It is expected that at the beginning of an intervention some families may experience resistance, anxiety, or fear of the unknown. Some people, however, may genuinely not like it and enjoy it, and therefore, fail to see any benefit. This is not a measure of you as a health practitioner; it might be the wrong time or even the wrong intervention for a particular person. In these cases, health practitioners are responsible of supporting these people to find something more suitable, for example support groups or individual therapy. Give them options which they can choose from.

Terminal Cancer and Bereavement

7.1 Prelude

Unexpectedly, my father got extremely sick while I was writing this book and passed away. I became the daughter of a father who was very ill. I knew some of the phases of this process from the literature, from talking to other people who had experienced this before me, but I was not ready for how I would feel, what I would think and how I would react. It was sad, sadness was everywhere in my body, in the house, in my thoughts, and that sadness remained ruling and untouchable for about two weeks, it dominated, until it dissipated and left space for peace to come in, for new to come in, for light to come in … and I welcomed them as best I could.

Even though I am old enough to understand death, I was never ready for my father to die. It was nothing like I could imagine, in fact it is something I think I'd rather never imagine, but it happened.

The first experience that I would like to share is that I was not close to my father and living through the expectations of others in terms of how I should be feeling and how sad I should be, was difficult. People have expectations about death that may or may not match your own, particularly those who were not even close to me had even more expectations of how sad I should be. So firstly, do not assume how a child feels when their parent dies, listen. But most importantly know that your perceptions and ideas may be different to theirs.

The death of a parent is ultimately a family event, an intimate family event that is dealt by the immediate family only, if families wish to, it can also include the extended family or friends. Ultimately families themselves need to make these decisions and need to be validated and supported in these decisions, not contradicted, not given advice unless requested. Knowing the person's wishes was fundamental, I am aware that these are difficult conversations to have and require a level of acceptance both from the ill parent and the family. At the time of deciding and processing, knowing what your parent wanted and sticking to their wishes provides comfort, but it is also the shield to all those comments and opinions from people that feel entitled to disagree. As a healthcare practitioner, suggesting the importance of this conversation is necessary, to offer and enable supports for this conversation to happen is fundamental. If families do not avail of the help, it is their right but they will remember that it was provided, and that will be respected.

Ideally, healthcare systems should be integrated, particularly in countries where a single health system exists. My father was a very sick person and towards his most critical time, several doctors were involved in his care. Days after he had passed away my mother kept getting phone call reminders of future appointments that he was no longer going to attend and these calls were very difficult for her to explain, very heart breaking to listen to as well. As a daughter I sometimes took the phone and finished the calls myself but as a healthcare practitioner I think they should have never happened. This is something we can do, inform other colleagues about the decease of our patient and the cancellation of appointments if they have access to this information, we can also just offer to do this for families ourselves or as part of a structured after bereavement supports for families. Ideally all hospitals, cancer care units should have dedicated people to continue and have an 'after death' check in with families. Again, families are entitled to avail of them or not.

I was back in college at the time of my father's illness and due to the COVID-19 pandemic I was also working remotely in Europe while living at home in Central America. Time of course was completely different, and many things were going on at strange times, literally and metaphorically. I was not the main carer of my father; I was one of the helpers only and usually the strongest one to pick him from the floor when he fainted or carried him up the stairs; when it was still possible for him to be there, upstairs, there was a point where it was not. He had an internal bleed now as well, I thought I might hurt him even more by putting him through the effort of the stairs but that was another battle lost, another moment where we knew he was not himself and he was becoming less and less himself.

I remembered at this time young people I met along my life who were main carers of their mothers and had to stop studying to mind their ill parent. I managed to continue but I understood how they could not. One night I was sitting with my computer on the two steps at the entrance to my house trying to submit the final assignment for one of my courses. The ambulance was parked in front of our house, it was almost midnight. Paramedics usually leave the ambulance running in case they need to drive away with the patient very quickly, so my mother asked me to stay downstairs to mind the ambulance. I sat there with my computer working on my assignment while my brain was 1,000 miles away. And yes, I know parental illness affects education and every aspect of a child and a young person's life, it was impossible to concentrate towards the end. One night my father fainted completely about 2:15 am, he fell to the floor and my sister, my mother and I ran as usual to try to get his blood pressure up, to make him more comfortable, I had an exam that same day at 3 am in the morning that I honestly did not have time to study for. I got a 75. At another time of my life, I would have been ashamed by a 75, that day at that time, that 75 was a miracle and still seems like it. Some people suggested that I should defer my exams, I didn't because I knew that if I got myself pass that line, I would be able to rest after, so I kept going. One of my lecturers found out that my father passed away because we had a meeting scheduled which I had to change for a week later. I needed to go on, to finish and then rest. That was my style, but I understand other people have different styles, different needs and all options should be provided for children and young people to make choices, their own choices based on how they feel, based on what they think they can do. Again, it is better to reject help than to not have it at all.

My mother, my sister and I planted a rose garden in honour of my father. We selected the colour of roses we liked and created a circle shape with them, eternity. I love it. My mother sends me photographs of the roses from time to time. It makes me happy. Bereavement is still an open process for me, I don't think the process is complete yet, but I can write about it and that gives me hope. I know families deserve their own rose gardens, happiness and hope, and this book is trying to help them find all three of them, with their favourite-coloured roses, with their favourite shapes and they can cut it in the shape and size they want.

Chapter Highlights

- Health practitioners need to reflect about their understanding/views on death. These can be different to those of children and families.
- Children and young people cope with parental terminal illness in many ways but overall, they should be informed and allowed to make their own decisions as early as possible.
- Parents need to be informed about the impact of treatments and how this will impact their children's lives so they can make informed decisions.
- More research is needed on how to support different families according to their composition and specific needs, for example single parent households.
- Family conflict is expected due to added stresses and demands.
- Current knowledge on the impact of parental death is conflictive, some identify difficulties such as stress, while others find children and young people have the capacity to adapt and do not present additional emotional or behavioural problems.
- Healthcare practitioners have a crucial role in supporting children and families, particularly in identifying unmet needs and support needs.

7.2   Understanding Death

One of the significant challenges that any practitioner may have is understanding bereavement. I suggest that before dealing with bereavement it is necessary to reflect on death and its personal meaning to you – what death is, what are the preconceptions of death we personally have and therefore how we can understand and empathise with somebody else going through the experience of death. More research is needed to fully understand how healthcare professionals and families can work together to adapt and cope at the time of parental cancer [125]. Research has described death as complex, challenging and an experience difficult to understand, particularly difficult to empathise with, as it can be very personal and unique. The way death is perceived depends on various factors including family structure, cultural background, personal beliefs, social support and social norms [125].

7.3 'Preparing' Children and Young People for Parental Death

This section describes ways in which research has suggested to support children when they find out the prognosis of their parent is death. Preparing is enclosed in speech marks because the death of a parent is and will be a difficult challenge for anyone, particularly for a child or young person. This can facilitate coping, but nothing can or will fully prepare a child or young person for losing a parent.

An interesting aspect, worth reflecting about the concept of 'preparing' at this point is the definition of it. What does it mean that a child is 'prepared' for the death of a parent? The term in research is used independent of this consideration and does not provide clear guidelines of how to ensure that a child is 'prepared' for the death of a parent and what this entails. Is this very 'personal' and unique or is it worth developing indicators that are mindful of children's cognitive and emotional development?

Children and families experiencing parental death from cancer are a vulnerable population, overlooked at times by healthcare professionals and researchers [29]. Despite this, research has provided some advice on how to improve the experience for children pre-bereavement [151]. These suggestions have been provided as generalisations and they may or may not be suitable for a particular young person. However, these can be offered as choices they can make and options which they may have not considered at the time that they may end up putting in practice.

Research and practice and palliative care have traditionally been an advocate for a client-centred approach [152] whereby interventions and supports are guided by the needs of the child or parent, and not solely by the criteria of an 'expert', practitioner. There are specific circumstances where practitioners will have to use their professional judgement to make decisions for a child or parent if their faculties or circumstances at the time imped them from doing so, for example they might be overwhelmed or in a lot of distress by the diagnosis to make difficult decisions. However, practitioners should always make decisions based on the needs of the children and families and ensure these correspond to their individual needs and characteristics. Check et al. [153], for example described that parents with advanced cancer may have difficulties planning for death and dying as well as advanced care planning. Knutsson et al. [112] propose a 'caring child-focused encounter', which is also holistic in nature, enabling practitioners to understand the child and how their surroundings are impacting them and identify their individual needs. The main objective is to 'include children more and forget them less' [112, p. 10]. This is not without its challenges and is impacted by parental and professional's beliefs, knowledge and fears.

Cancer can be changing and uncertain, therefore providing a precise estimate of when parental death will finally occur can be challenging [151]. Despite this, it is crucial that healthcare practitioners inform parents and provide clear information regarding declining health conditions and terminal cancer diagnoses as early as possible as this will enable parents to prepare their children and young people for the impending death [151, 154].

Despite the conceptual complexity of death, research has provided evidence of the consequences that children 'less prepared' for parental death may experience including hostility, resentment, guilt and anxiety [151]. Children, over 7 years of age, can experience fears of making their parent more ill by bringing external germs or viruses, fear of upsetting their parents with their questions or their own health concerns and fears of losing their parent in their lives [155]. Parental terminal cancer can also lead to other challenges for children including witnessing the secondary effects of the treatments and seeing their parent ill or suffering [155]. The impact of side effects can be greater in children (8–18 years) who fulfilled a caring role for their ill parent and their families [155]. Regarding symptoms Kennedy and Lloyd-Williams [155] have suggested that children and young people would benefit from having more accurate information about the treatment and its effects, for example no effects may not necessarily mean 'good health' and increased physical symptoms may not mean 'bad' health [155]. This might help reduce children's anxiety or confusion about cancer and treatment side effects.

Another aspect to be aware of as healthcare practitioners is that children and young people have different ways of coping with parental terminal cancer [155]. Therefore, there isn't a single or correct way to deal. Some of the strategies used by children and young people identified by research include:

- Reasoning.
- Having a positive attitude such as listening to uplifting stories from friends or the media.
- Having or looking for facts and information.
- Continue with their normal activities.
- Maintaining normality.
- Distraction (taking the mind off things, spending time with friends or in social activities).
- Talking (or not talking) about it.
- Maximising time with their ill parent.
- Faith.

Stressful experiences such as parental death can activate attachment proximity seeking in children. This means that the availability of a figure who they are attached to can help to reduce their fear, establish normal routines and act as a biological and behavioural regulator [157]. Parental death for young children means the loss of an important attachment figure which can be 'inherently traumatic' for them as young children are usually very dependent on this carer and rely on them for self-regulation and to carry out daily routines and activities [157]. Therefore, young children may benefit from having physical contact with their parents. Research has provided several recommendations on how to support children and young people [152, 156]:

- Children and young people should be given the choice to be with their parent at the time of their death.

- Strengthening the child or young person's relationship with the surviving caregiver through positive reinforcement and supportive communication can create a sense of routine and consistency for the child.

- Children and young people should have access to information about the nature of their parent's illness and the potential outcome.

- Some young people may benefit from keeping normality and routines; however, others may benefit from distractions from the intense situation they are experiencing.

- Spending time with friends and peers is a developmental characteristic of young people; however, it can also be important at this time as a distraction and/or as a source of support.

Even though it is less researched, parental terminal cancer can also have a positive impact in children and young people's lives. This includes, for example learning how to care for others, increased independence, learning about priorities, being more prepared for adult life and a higher appreciation for their parent and family [155]. Some children described that parental illness had also brought their families closer together [155]. These positive interactions seem to be helpful for children and young people post-bereavement [155].

7.4 Parental and Family[1] Coping

A terminal cancer diagnosis for any parent with children and young people has been described in the literature as a highly stressful event [151]. A diagnosis of this nature can evoke anxiety, depression and parental distress which may impact on their parenting and family relationships [154]. Furthermore, the psychological distress associated with a parental diagnosis of advanced cancer may have long lasting effects and continue into adulthood [155].

---

[1] Family in this book is used as a comprehensive term to include different types and compositions of families.

At the time of a terminal cancer diagnosis, parents who have dependent children experience more distress than non-parents, particularly regarding communicating with their children about the disease [6, 12]. Having a child has an impact on the type of cancer care patients select and the decisions they make. Some parents prioritise the extension of life so that they can spend more time with their children, other parents instead chose to preserve their physical condition to remain physically close to their children and continue with their parenting responsibilities for as long as possible [153]. Therefore, families have different priorities, and this will impact their decision-making, which will consequently impact the children and young people. Regarding support at this crucial time, research has found that parents rarely discuss their parental identity and how this fits with their treatment preferences with their oncology team [149]. This can lead to a discrepancy between treatment demands, schedules and effects compared with parents' ideas of effective parenting which may lead to a lack of adherence to treatment and emotional distress in parents [149]. Therefore, healthcare practitioners need to make sure parents are allowed to speak about their concerns and are allowed to make decisions about treatment with knowledge of the impact this will have on children and young people.

The experience of terminal illness and bereavement is shaped by family characteristics, including family cohesion and communication. More open communication, for example can make children feel more valued, less lonely and less anxious [151]. Healthcare professionals have been identified as having a key role in providing communication guidance for parents with cancer [12]. The need for empathy and understanding towards parents has also been identified as crucial. Professionals need to acknowledge the challenges and difficulties of a parent diagnosed with terminal cancer [12] to acknowledge the importance of providing guidance and support, or at least to offer it, whether it is received or not is important that parents are empowered and informed about possible supports they can access if needed and desired.

The capacity to support children and families initially through a terminal cancer diagnosis and bereavement is determined by the attitude of the family towards the diagnosis. Research has found that many parents decide not to communicate the prognosis to their children to protect them. This, however, can mean that children are less prepared to deal with parental death and may be exposed to more adversity as a result [151, 158]. A similar study carried out with young people between 11 and 26 years of age also found that withholding information can result on a lack of awareness about the seriousness of the illness and delayed the identification of support needs and accessing these supports [159].

Research has found an important challenge in potentially supporting children and families at this time which is the discrepancy between the needs expressed by children and how parents perceive them and validate them (or not). This can impact children's ability to ask for help and access it. Kennedy [155] found that parents acknowledged the impact of cancer on children, whereas others believed that their children were not impacted by parental illness and emphasised the need for 'normality' and did not have open communication with their children. Children who openly spoke about their illness were described by their parents as coping better if they supported open communication, whereas those who were in favour of closed communication perceived children who were quieter as coping better [155]. Parents also expressed feelings of pride to their children according to the way they coped, suggesting that parents reinforce and shape the way children cope [155]. Therefore, practitioners need to understand parents' views as these will impact on their perception of whether a child may need support or not. Research has encouraged age-appropriate communication between parents and children and there is evidence to support the benefits of this. The patient and their families, however, are entitled to decide which information regarding their diagnosis and prognosis is shared [160] with children and young people. Healthcare practitioners need to ensure that parents and families have enough information to make informed decisions about themselves and their families.

Knutsson et al. [112] found that nurses, in their study, had to encourage parents to understand the benefit for children visiting the ill parent. Parents had to be motivated by talking to them about why it is important to allow a child to see what is really happening, as this stops them from imagining worse situations in their minds and it helps them feel included. When these physical visits are not possible, the situation can be made more visible to the child by taking photographs, for example [112]. Children need to be supported when they are in the hospital setting; practitioners can do this by using the following strategies [112]:

- Meet the child in the waiting room and explain to them what the room environment will be like, for example if other patients will be in the room as well.
- Reassure the child that they will be able to manage the situation.
- Walk with the child to the room and do not leave them alone.
- Show the child the equipment and explain to them what it does and how it works.
- Include a follow-up meeting to ensure the child or young person is doing well after the experience.

An important aspect to consider as well is to ensure that the child or young person can decide whether they are interested in taking this tour themselves and facilitate this for the child and their specific needs.

Length of the disease, and how long children and young people must adapt to it, is an indicator of how long they must 'prepare' for parental death. Bereaved adolescents tend to experience higher levels of maladaptive coping strategies than those whose parents survived cancer [7]. Time, however, seems to be a determinant of coping strategies since lengthy disease duration has been linked with poor adjustment but also with better adjustment as young people have more time to acclimatise to the illness. Those who experience cancer for a shorter period may have little time to enact coping strategies [7]. Adolescents need to be given more space, physically and psychologically to reduce feelings of intrusiveness [112].

Research has described that most parents want to reduce the impact of their illness in their children to the maximum possible [155]. Parents, however, recognised that children can experience changes in their daily routines and social activities, for example helping around the house and carrying out other chores such as shopping [155].

Terminally ill parents may have several concerns at this challenging time. Bugge et al. [154] identified some of the needs and concerns which terminally ill parents have. These are:

- Need for reassurance and confirmation that they are supporting their children and not causing any harm or trauma to them.

- Parents need help starting conversations about the future to prepare the family at a time of impending death.

- Parents appreciated 'child-friendly' environments in health settings as this enabled the presence of their children at the time of dying/death.

- Parents also wanted opportunities to create memories with their children.

Support provision for families is also impacted by availability and access to support services. This will facilitate or limit the family's capacity to request and receive support at critical times where they may benefit from additional supports from practitioners on how to explain death and bereavement to their children [151]. Research has highlighted that it is almost a universal practice that healthcare professionals advocate for open communication about the illness in families; however, mechanisms and supports need to exist as parents should not be left feeling accountable and at the same time unprepared and anxious to be able to achieve the task of open communication [12].

Parental terminal cancer can impact different families in different ways. To organise these differences, Park et al. [161] provided a profile of families based on their reactions to terminal cancer. What is particularly interesting about these profiles are the differences regarding their will to get support, both formal and informal. Some families would therefore be more open to be supported than others. Families with more complex dynamics may also require more complex interventions and supports [161]. Table 7.1 describes the type of families and coping and communication styles, highlighting the difference between prepared and less prepared families [161].

Table 7.1 Family types and communication patterns

Pattern	Family description
Prepared and optimistic	Personally optimistic and hopeful.
	Expecting minimal illness burden or disease remission in the future.
	Confidence in capacity to manage their parental role and illness.
	Article I. Open to receive informal supports from social networks.
	Article II. Open to receive professional support.
	Article III. Fear of missing out on their children's lives but still enjoy family time.
Equipped and pragmatic	Fear about the illness progression and changes in their parental roles.
	Believed that the illness led to psychological distress in their children.
	Article IV. Perceived that they and their children were successfully adapting to the illness, even though they had mild to moderate symptoms.
	Article V. Prioritised family relationships and were accepting and adapting to the illness.
	Article VI. Open to informal and professional support.
Discouraged and struggling	Reported substantially greater illness impact and psychological distress. Most were unable to carry out normal work activities and spent long hours of rest which did not allow them to carry out parental responsibilities.
	Proactive in their communication with their children.
Apprehensive and passive	Mixed views of their illness and its impact.
	Concerned about dying before the children reached adulthood.
	Article VII. Some experienced difficult marital relationships before and/or after the illness.
	Article VIII. These parents tried to normalise and minimise the impact of the illness and did not discuss the seriousness of the illness with their children.
	Parents used informal supports but were not interested in seeking professional supports.
Discouraged and conflicted	Feeling discouraged, experiencing substantial functional difficulties and unable to manage their parental duties due to the illness and the effects of treatment.
	Acknowledged their prognosis and how their children would not have them in the future.
	These were usually single parents with poor relationships with the child's biological parents or were married with little parent–couple quality relationships.
	Adopted a 'compressed' approach to parenting to prepare their children as a legacy, however, did not engage in discussions about the illness.
	Parents used informal supports and had looked for professional supports regarding concerns with their family issues.

7.5 Family Support Programmes

Even though cancer research has focused on the impact of parental cancer on the family, the research with different family styles and compositions is very limited. It has been highlighted that the needs of children may vary when considering the composition of their families. Children from divorced or separated families may change the current living situation for children and this needs to be discussed and agreed between the dying and the healthy parent, as well as with the children or young people in the family [154]. Family-based supports have been described in the literature as an alternative to support families when a parent has a diagnosis of terminal cancer.

Bugge et al. [154] designed and evaluated a family support programme underpinned by Family Resilience Theory. The programme focused on three main components: reframe the crisis by talking about the illness, help parents understand the needs of their children to increase support within the family and plan for their future. This programme was delivered in a Norwegian hospital but what was most significant about it is that, as the programme was hospital based, families who were provided with a terminal cancer diagnosis were invited to the programme.

Hospital-based programmes have the advantage that children, young people and families who require or may require supports are already identified and therefore the provision of support can begin in a timely manner [162]. Additionally, the hospital is already a familiar environment for patients which may motivate their willingness to engage in supports and to bring their children and young people into a context that is already familiar to them. It may also reduce the extra burden for patients to find services outside the hospital, which may require some degree of research or knowledge to be able to identify them, access them, trust them and in general just for families to navigate their way through a new organisation or a new environment.

Family support programmes need to be aware and adaptable to be able to capture and embrace the different needs of families. Families have a common underlying experience of parental terminal cancer; however, they are unique in their makeup, dynamics, concerns and circumstances [150]. Family needs must be assessed and dealt with to ensure families are getting the support they need. Family-based interventions targeted at enhancing parents' ability to meet the needs of their children particularly their need for emotional support, physical care and open communication have been identified as effective [163].

7.6 Family Conflict

Family conflict can be present at the end-of-life stage [164]. Several factors can lead to conflict, for example families being and feeling unprepared for the intense demands of home care (managing symptoms, managing care, pain control, personal caregiving, bathing, feeding, toileting) and the emotional impact of the dying process, while balancing multiple life responsibilities [164]. Additionally, there can be several factors outside the family which can contribute to end-of-life conflict. These include societal expectations and norms, communication problems (e.g. missed opportunities for early discussion, avoidance of difficult conversations), gaps in legal issues as well as the perception of death [164].

Kramer and Boelk [164] gathered different suggestions to support families when conflict occurs. These are:

- Separate people and relationship issues from the actual problem.
- Focus on interests and benefits for all parties.
- Create solutions by brainstorming with the family. Invite questions that promote reflection and curiosity.
- Acknowledge the strengths of the family.
- Recur to objective criteria and facts to support the best course of action, scientific facts or legal recommendations.

7.7   The Impact of Parental Death

The impact of parental cancer can be determined by a variety of factors, individual developmental factors including age and gender and other contextual factors such as family functioning and family communication [18]. This section will provide a description of the impact of parental death on children and young people; however, it is important to highlight that the precision of this information is limited by the evidence available. Studies usually include a wide variety of ages under the same label of children which may include different developmental stages, levels of maturity and developmental needs which may vary within those subgroups.

Research has identified some of the 'common' or expected reactions of children within the first two years after the death happened [157]. One of the limitations, however, is the way in which it is presented, as the data is not presented according to age or developmental stage but under a common term 'child'. These reactions identified included dysphoria, depression, generalised anxiety, separation anxiety and posttraumatic stress. Dealing with the physical absence of the deceased parent is not the only challenge for bereaved children. These children may have also been exposed to potentially traumatic images and situations associated with the death and therefore increasing the likelihood of developing posttraumatic symptoms [156]. The death of a primary caregiver may also bring disruption in the child's sense of security and sense of self [157].

The impact of death from cancer in a parent can be stressful and potentially traumatic for children and young people. For this reason, it should be considered a relevant public health issue [156, 163]. MacPherson and Emelus [162] have highlighted the need for education in the field of death and bereavement particularly in the community, regarding how to respond to a bereaved child or parent, as a lack of information and understanding is prevalent.

Research findings regarding the impact of parental death are conflicting, some studies suggesting that young people experiencing parental cancer experience more difficulties, such as stress, compared with young people whose parents survived a cancer diagnosis [154, 165] and have described the experience as traumatic particularly without appropriate supports [156, 158]. Other studies, however, did not find that children that experience parental death had additional emotional or behavioural problems compared with children who were experiencing parental cancer in other disease stages [18]. Due to these conflicting findings, it is important to assume or pathologise a child only because they have experienced parental death, research has instead found that children and young people have the capacity to adapt [152]. It has been suggested that only a small number of children (5–10%) in the general population experience clinically significant psychiatric problems [157].

Another aspect which has not been thoroughly explored is parent's preference for place of dying and the impact this has on children and young people. This is a topic of concern for parents as some may believe that a death at home will expose the children [153]. Engaging in palliative care is an alternative to home dying; however, some patients may be unclear about what palliative care is and how they might benefit from it [153]. Comparative studies carried out with children experiencing parental cancer or parental death identified that those experiencing bereavement had higher level of posttraumatic stress symptoms, however, both cohorts were reporting similar levels of anxiety and depression [156]. This suggests that parental death and parental illness pose different challenges to children but also may share similarities in terms of the impact both events.

Research carried out specifically with young people found that post-bereavement, the level of distress and unidentified needs was associated with individual factors, such as age and gender, and not by whether young people had support pre-bereavement [159]. Older young people may experience more distress at pre-bereavement because they have a better understanding of the prognosis of parental cancer, they can also, however, articulate their need for support and access services themselves, whereas younger ones may only seek for support if prompted to do so [159].

It is important to consider that not all young people experience emotional and behavioural problems. Kennedy [155] has highlighted that there is a need for additional research in the field of parental advanced cancer. Evidence so far suggests that the period of parental terminal illness may be a more difficult period for children than the time after parental death. Kuhne et al. [18] carried out a study in Germany with 86 young people between 11 and 21 years of age. This study compared young people experiencing parental palliative care and those experiencing parental cancer at different disease stages. The study found that young people whose parents were in palliative care had significantly less emotional and behavioural problems and better quality of life than those young people with parents in other cancer stages. It is also important to consider that

Kuhne et al. [18] did not find significant differences by adolescent's age or gender. This study, however, included a cohort made up of a convenience sample of middle and upper social class families that were already engaging with a counselling service. Young people, within the two years after parental death has occurred may experience depressive symptoms [157]. It is important to consider that children may have individual strengths and difficulties which may result in a different experience for each child. One of these differences identified is in coping styles. Howell et al. [156] found that coping styles in children (7–13 years) was associated with their level of reported posttraumatic stress, anxiety and depression [157].

7.8 Bereavement

Central to this chapter is the awareness that the process of bereavement can lead to significant changes in people's usual behaviours, thoughts and emotions. This is expected to an extent as experiencing the death of somebody loved has been defined as a challenging and devastating experience [64]. This chapter intentionally excludes the term 'normal' to refer to bereavement; as the evidence is clear in suggesting that bereavement is a unique, individual process and practitioners will be dealing with a series of 'normalities', as varied as the individuals that experience bereavement themselves, that is every child or young person will deal with bereavement in their own way, even within the same family unit. Cultural and developmental variation may also impact differently on children and young people's bereavement processes [157]. This can pose a challenge for a practitioner to identify what is part of their bereavement process, and what is now placing the child or young person at risk. Bereavement reactions need to be understood in the cultural, religious, family traditions, personality and age norms of the context [157, 166].

The impact of parental death and children's ability to cope is heavily related to the environment and how facilitating it may be [157]. The environment can also facilitate or inhibit a child's ability to cope with bereavement [157]. A death in the family can have adverse consequences such as inhibiting family practices and inability to maintain positive interactions between children and their parents [157]. Other circumstances can also impact negatively on children and young people including financial strain, home relocations or loss of health insurance because of parental death [157]. Surviving parents and caregivers can help children and adolescents cope by establishing positive family routines, warmth and good communication between parents and children [157].

7.9 How to Support Children and Young People

The role of practitioners becomes particularly important regarding the unmet needs of children and young people experiencing parental cancer. These needs are support and understanding, help with coping with feelings, talking to people with similar experiences, information, having a break, space, time to grieve and help with household responsibilities [163]. These unmet needs can help inform the design and objectives of any support services targeted at children and young people to ensure services are targeted to and respond to their needs.

Opportunities need to be provided for children and young people to be able to express themselves. Avoiding discussion about emotions or recurring to denial of emotions may place a young person in a very vulnerable position as they will not have access to supports and this may increase their feelings of loneliness, isolation and anxiety [163]. Children need to be helped to identify their needs but also to be able to communicate them to others, particularly others who can support them if needed [162]. This aspect is important, according to MacPherson [162], as children need empathy and benefit from making a connection with somebody who understands them, somebody they can relate to and make them feel like they are understood. Research has also reported that parents acknowledge that their children might need another person to speak to, besides the surviving parent [162], but did not always feel capable of accessing these supports [155]. Practitioners can fulfil this role; however, there must be a relationship, a connection between the child and the practitioner, which may require some time or effort to be developed.

Practitioners need to be willing to spend this time and effort and ensure that children and young people are receptive of the support being provided. Research has found that practitioners need to be engaged and motivated to enable the process of involving children, as they act as the 'gatekeepers' that allow the child into the hospital and support them during and after the visit to their parent [112]. Some practitioners, however, may feel inadequately prepared to discuss the topic with parents [6].

The current literature has identified several ways in which children and young people deal with grief from parental death. Can Teen Australia [166, 167], a specialised support service for young people experiencing cancer in their families enumerated a list of possible ways in which grief can be expressed. Some of these were: wanting to be alone, talking, being silent, laughing, throwing things out, wanting to change address, not wanting to change anything in the house, talking to the deceased, listening to a song, engaging in activities that they used to do together among others. What is interesting about this list is the fact that it is long, but it also includes completely opposite behaviours that may be experienced by the same person at different times. Therefore, practitioners need to be aware that children and young people may express their grief in several ways which can also change over time. Some children may need time and space to 'escape' from the intensity of the situation of parental death and to work through their grief [152]. This escape also came in the form of keeping routine and normality, as it was a source of security and stability [152].

Research has shown that accessing peer support is an unmet need of young people [163]. For this reason, young people may benefit from the skills to access supports from other peers who may have also experienced parental death. These programmes could include the development of skills such as emotional awareness, express feelings constructively, listening skills, empathy, problem solving, stress management and assertiveness [163]. It is important to also consider the safety of young people engaging with peers. It may be necessary to create face-to-face or online environments where young people can express themselves safely and where mechanisms are in place to support them if they become upset. A possibility is to create support groups led by adult, trained practitioners to act as gatekeepers and to invite young people to the group and deal with issues of Child Safety and consent to take part in the group. The groups themselves do not have to be run by adults, instead this may be an opportunity to let young people facilitate their own group or train adolescents who have experienced parental cancer in the past to support other young people who are going through the experience at the time. An appropriate and safe environment should also be considered.

Another source of social support can be school. Schools have been identified as crucial environments for children and young people who experience bereavement, as they spend a significant amount of their time in school. The school can be a very negative experience for children and young people if the right mechanisms are not in place. MacPherson and Emelus [152] found that schools were very important environments, but issues emerged when schools lacked the policies, the communication mechanisms and teachers did not have the understanding on the topic. To prevent these issues in schools, research has suggested that school-based psycho-education programmes can be beneficial to help students and school staff to gain understanding and awareness of the challenges that young people experience when they have lost a parent [163]. These programmes can also provide information about grief that normalise the experience for students who may experience grief themselves and are concerned about seeming different to their peers. Knowledge on death and bereavement should be included in the school curriculum [152].

Supporting children and families can be challenging for practice; however, research has identified some facilitators that may enable this process [64].

1. Developing early rapport. Building relationships with parents from the time of diagnosis has been identified as key to facilitate connections with children and parents.

2. Consider parental wishes and decisions. Practitioners need to ensure that the voices of parents are heard; this will contribute to build a relationship of trust and will provide practitioners access to the children and young people. This relationship will also allow parents to encourage parents to talk to their children, allowing them to visit the parent and be involved in parental care.

Practitioners can provide support for children and young people by helping them make informed choices and be aware of their 'rights'. Canteen [166, p. 10] provided a list of these rights which may be useful to share with children and young people and support them to have these rights met:

- Access information and obtain answers for their questions.
- Grieve in any way they wish as long as it is safe for them and people around them.
- Keep their thoughts and emotions to themselves.
- Feel anger towards the deceased parent, life, the situation, etc.
- Not follow other people's expectations of how they should grief or cope.
- Have their own beliefs and understanding of death.
- Have their own rituals to support their bereavement process, for example punch a pillow, exercise, watch a sad movie, listen to music, writing down their thoughts and emotions, call a helpline, walk the dog, etc..
- Talk about the deceased (if they wish to do so).
- Laugh and have fun while grieving.
- Learn to live with the death and get on with their lives.

Practitioners, however, can also face barrier when supporting children and families. Families' wishes and decisions can be a barrier for practitioner support provision. Some families may choose not to disclose information about the severity of parental illness and eventual death. Some parents may be in 'denial' of the situation, and this limits practitioner's capacity to provide support [64]. Children may also be 'invisible', meaning that they are not allowed to visit their parents in hospital or in a hospice, or may not be present when practitioners carry out home visits or might deliberately refuse to engage [64]. This will make it difficult to contact children and being able to identify if they need support and how best to support them.

7.10 Signs of Additional Need

The literature suggests that bereaved children need specially targeted interventions, as their needs are different those children with non-life-threatening diagnoses [17]. One of the biggest challenges practitioners have is identifying when changes in behaviours, emotions and thoughts are no longer part of the natural process of coping with the loss but may instead place a child or young person in a situation of risk, vulnerability or danger. This chapter will provide an account of the evidence currently available to understand bereavement and its effects but also to identify children and young people who may be at risk. It is important to highlight that the current findings do not provide a definite solution for this issue of where and how to 'draw the line' between bereavement reactions and risk behaviours.

One of the first discrepancies identified in the literature is related with duration. The definition of the Adjustment Disorder Related to Bereavement criteria included in the DSM-5 Diagnostic and Statistical Manual of Mental Disorders (5th Edition) stipulates a period of one year after the death has occurred as the time needed to consider it as an adjustment disorder, whereas other sources [157] suggest that this time should be reduced to six months as children who may experience pathological bereavement will do so in the first months. There are also developmental reasons for this – one year can mean a major developmental period for a child and therefore a potentially lost opportunity for early intervention [151].

Kaplow et al. [157] provided guidelines to identify bereavement-related disorders in children and young people to identify when behaviours, attitude and emotions are not part of a person's bereavement process. One of the major limitations of this model and criteria provided by Kaplow et al. [157] is that there are no guidelines on the number of symptoms required to suggest the presence of a possible disorder. The components of this model are described below:

1. **Persistent yearning or longing for the deceased**

Toddlers and very young children, due to developmental reason, may lack the concept of permanence of death and experience separation distress or reuniting fantasies; this may be evident in their behaviours such as talking to the person on a toy phone [157]. Young children may return to the where they last saw the deceased as an expression of their longing [157].

2. **Intense sorrow or emotional pain**

Young children may struggle to verbalise their sadness, but this can be identified in their play patterns as well as anxiety when they separate from their carers, anger and withdrawal [157].

3. **Preoccupation with the person who died**

In small children this preoccupation can be expressed as their need to sleep in the deceased person's bed, wearing their clothes, preoccupation regarding the circumstances of the death or re-enactment of the death through play. Children may also experience repetitive fantasies of how they could have prevented the death [157].

4. **Difficulty accepting the death**

According to Kaplow et al. [157] finding it difficult to accept the death can be normal for children and young people, particularly those under five years of age, due to their cognitive inability to understand the permanence of death. Older children and adolescents may need an external caregiver to confirm the death and to support them in their bereavement process.

5. **Anger related to the loss**

Anger in children and young people may be expressed as irritability, tantrums, oppositional behaviour and conduct problems in response to changes in their daily routine. This may also be linked to others enacting the deceased parent role [157].

6. Maladaptive appraisals of the self

These maladaptive appraisals are usually identified in adolescents, for example they may believe that somebody else is responsible for the death. They may also perceive that they are blamed for the death by other people [157].

7. Excessive avoidance of reminders of loss

Research has found that excessive avoidance is a predictor of functional impairment [157].

8. Social identity disruptions

Children and young people may express a desire not to live as they wish to be with the deceased. In adolescents, this can include suicidal ideation, careless behaviours, risk-taking behaviours and drug abuse [157].

9. Difficulty trusting other people

After the death, children may struggle to establish relationships with new caregivers and may be involved in oppositional or defiant behaviours [157].

10. Feeling alone or detached

Children and young people may feel alone or detached from others as they feel 'different' to their peers who have not experienced the death. Children may feel alone in their grief particularly if they are having difficulties such as experiencing connections with the deceased (thinking they have seen them or heard them). Adolescents may conceal their grief to protect the surviving parent and avoid emotional strain on them [157].

11. Life is meaningless or empty

Children and young people may feel their lives are empty or meaningless without the deceased and that they cannot function with their deceased parent. Research has found it challenging to determine how a young child may express this, but it might be expressed through behaviours such as lethargy, withdrawal, lack of interest in situations, people, or places which they enjoyed before. Children may also show developmental regressions, new fears and disruption in their eating and sleeping patterns [157]. In adolescents, this may be expressed in a lack of interest to form age-appropriate aspirations such as career choices and family life.

12. Role and identity confusion

Children and adolescents may experience shame or embarrassment associated with parental death, this is a unique experience that their peers may not understand. They may experience a loss in their competence and their ability to do things without the support of the deceased parent. Role confusion may be caused by having additional responsibilities or having to assume more adult-like roles because of parental death, which may include a caring role for younger siblings, for example [157]. Children may also experience excessive worry for their surviving caregiver or other family members.

13. Health

Grief can also manifest as physical symptoms including weight loss or gain, headaches, altered sleeping patterns, exhaustion, body aches and pains, stomach upsets, lack of breath, colds, infections, elevated heart rate and dizziness [166]. It is important to consider these symptoms as over time they may have a significant impact on children and adolescent health.

Treasure Box [63]

You know what I did the other day? I made my own personal treasure box! Mum and I got a shoebox and we decorated it with colourful things. We decided that the box was going to be full of things that make me happy and smile.

On the outside we stuck pictures cut out from magazines of things that were brightly coloured. I said that rainbows made me happy, so we only chose pictures of things that were the colours of the rainbow. My box looked so bright and funky once we had done it.

Next, we filled the box with all my treasures! We put photos from the family album in and tickets from the cinema because we went to see a really funny film the other day. I found a beautiful feather on a walk the other day and put that in my box too. We also wrote down nice words about each other and about those inside the box.

Note: A variation of the treasure box has been used for working with bereavement for children and young people. Treasure boxes can be used to store happy memories and happy moments lived with the dead parent which the child/young person wants to remember forever.

7.11   Implications for Practice

- Children and young people require psychosocial support at every stage of parental illness, as this is a critical life event that may lead to distress at every stage not only at terminal stages of parental cancer [168].

- Services to support children and families should be 'client-centred', having the needs of children and families as the priority, based on their individual needs.

- Having a child advocate or a child representative with sole responsibility of supporting children and young people and focusing on their needs will ensure that the experience for children is improved [112].

- The views of bereaved children and families should be included in the development of interventions and services, to ensure these reflect the real needs of children and families [146].

- Families may benefit from psychoeducational materials and information focused on how to identify early signs of distress and a heightened risk of developing posttraumatic stress or maladaptive grief [156].

- Integrating support services for families into patient's medical and palliative care treatments can be beneficial [154].

- More education and awareness about the needs of bereaved children and families need to be provided at a community level, at home and in school to ensure these needs are being met [162]. These issues may need to be also approached in policy [162].

- Families at the end-of-life benefit from routine screening for the early identification and prevention of conflict [164]. Standardised tools can contribute to this. Some suggested tools are Family Relationship Index [169], The Family Conflict at the End of Life (FC-EOL) scale [164].

- There is a need to normalise death, generating comfort around topics such as death and dying can help reduce family conflict, communication constraints and life-sustaining options [158]. Health practitioners can have a crucial role in this by normalising death, coordinating early referrals to hospice and addressing family needs throughout the process of care [164].

Self-Care for Practitioners

8.1   Introduction

Welcome to the last chapter of this book. I sincerely wanted this book to become a tool to support healthcare practitioners in their work with parents, children and families. I am aware that the book includes a lot of information, and you are at least overwhelmed at this stage. So, the idea of including this chapter at the end is to acknowledge the fact that working in the field of cancer is rewarding (that is why I do it) but it can also be overwhelming. Cancer is a challenging, difficult, scary story with a happy ending, most of the time, but it can lead to suffering, sadness and even death in some cases. I have cried many times and I think many more times are still to come. What I am trying to say is that I know this is hard and therefore you need to take care of yourself to keep supporting others because physical, mental and emotional burden will happen at some stage of your career or even of your day. This chapter is to support YOU.

I have included a list of implications for practice at the end of every chapter, some, or most of them are asks and demands on you, I know that also. As a health practitioner there are many expectations and responsibilities on you and working with families, children and young people who experience parental cancer adds an extra layer of responsibilities and demands. Research has suggested that healthcare practitioners have the duty to meet the needs of patients and their families; however, it has also been described that some practitioners lack the skills and knowledge to meet these needs themselves. Resources include personal resources as well as more structural ones [170].

I have emphasised this, parental cancer is a 'family business' and healthcare practitioners should respond accordingly, considering the needs of all members of the family, responding in age-appropriate ways. The ask on you is big; therefore, I hope this chapter will help YOU cope with all those responsibilities and expectations as well as any other personal challenges you may have. Overall, this chapter includes many suggestions, but only some may work for you. Please try them but most of all, make a commitment with yourself on how you will begin to or improve the ways in which you are already taking care of yourself.

8.2 Self-Care to Care for Others

Research has found that healthcare practitioners in general, and particularly those involved in oncology and palliative care may experience distress and grief associated with suffering in their patients and experiences of loss and unprocessed grief. This can compromise a person's well-being and lead to burnout, moral distress, compassion fatigue and potentially poor clinical decisions that can negatively impact patient care [171].

Self-care can be defined as the activities individually performed to promote and maintain personal well-being through the life course, minimise burnout, compassion fatigue and moral distress [169]. Self-care can also enhance job engagement expressed as efficacy, energy and involvement at work. Compassion satisfaction can also be increased as the pleasure of helping others and resilience can be increased as the ability to respond positively to challenging experiences [169]. Overall self-care can bring gratification and a sense of personal purpose.

8.3 Understanding Your Own Needs

The same way I have explained in earlier chapters, individuality and uniqueness is important in families and children, but this is also important for healthcare practitioners. We are all different, we have strong qualities and weaker ones, and we have different needs and ways to meet them. Golsater et al. [170] identified a profile of nurses according to their perception of the role they have in supporting children whose parents have a serious illness (see Table 8.1). These categories can be applied to other healthcare professions. They are not exhaustive, and not a judgement, so should not try to fit into one of them; this might help you understand yourself; that is all I would like this to be used for.

Table 8.1 Profile of healthcare professionals

Category	Definition
Being convinced it is not the nurse's responsibility	1. Focus on patient care and not on other family members (including children). 2. Contact with children is very limited as they are not present in the unit; children's place is in school and not visiting the parent in hospital. 3. Professionals should not interfere, and families should decide for themselves. 4. They lack the resources and skills to take care of children and believe they have nothing to offer.
Parents have the responsibility for the child's health	1. Parents are responsible for their children's health when one parent is in hospital, however, there is a recognition that parents may be exhausted, feeling guilty and are not always able to meet the child's needs. 2. Practitioners should show that children are welcome and state the benefits of involving the child.
Others can help the children	1. Other professionals are in a better position to support the children. These professionals usually coordinate contacts or referrals to other professionals, psychologists, counsellors or the child's school. 2. There is a perception that society fails to adequately support children as relatives.
Unable to fulfil the responsibility to care for children	1. Professionals feel responsible for caring for children but are unable to fulfil this obligation. 2. Children do not visit the unit often and staff do not meet them. 3. Units may have a child advocate who takes care of the children, but professionals may not feel that they have the knowledge, experience and fear. 4. Professionals welcome advice from the counsellors as to how to deal with the child.
Acknowledging children as relatives at the unit	1. Acknowledge children and want the encounter to be natural. 2. Children are allowed to visit their parents and can see the equipment. 3. Staff want to create a relationship with the child in a natural and easy manner.
Working systematically to fulfil the needs of children as relatives and involving them	Provide care in a structured manner. Children are allowed to be involved in parental care, considering their level of maturity. Information is provided to children with brochures, pamphlets and literature.

8.4   The Impact of Supporting Children and Families on Practitioners

This chapter began with the premise that supporting children and families is difficult and can have an emotional burden for practitioners [2, 64, 170]. This, however,
should not be a reason to be discouraged from doing it, but it instead highlights the
need to have facilitators and mechanisms in place to facilitate the support provi-
sions and reduce the challenges and emotional impact on practitioners.

Research has suggested that supporting children and families can be a significant emotional investment for practitioners, particularly those who may
lack formal training, which may also mean that practitioners are reluctant to
engage or may fear causing damage to a child or family [158]. Research has
also suggested that the worst situation has already happened for children and
young people when they get a diagnosis of parental cancer, particularly a terminal diagnosis, therefore silence may be counterproductive instead [4].

Oncology settings can be stressful, and staff can be at a risk of compassion
fatigue and burnout [172]. Working in oncology can be emotionally intense
due to repeatedly witnessing loss, death, physical and emotional pain, in cancer
patients and families as well as being confronted with their own mortality and
of their loved ones [166]. Practitioners expressed concern about their capacity
to remain professional when the nature of the issue is so emotional, and they
expressed wanting emotional support to deal with this [2].

8.5   Understanding Compassion Fatigue and Burnout

Oncology work can place healthcare practitioners at a heightened risk of compassion fatigue and burnout [172]. Research with health and social care professionals supporting parents and dependent children [64] has shown that
personal emotions can have an impact on professional behaviours, and this can
enhance or inhibit a practitioner's ability to connect empathically with parents
and children. This can lead to significant issues and formal diagnosis, for example compassion fatigue and burnout.

Compassion fatigue is defined as 'overexposure to suffering and pain that can
cause personal stress and a reduced ability to be empathetic' [172, p. 771]. It is also
known as 'the cost of caring' [173, p. 778]. The stress associated with compassion
fatigue is related to the wish of relieving a person from their suffering, which when
exceeded, can lead to symptoms including frustration, irritability, tension, sadness, withdrawal, numbness, emotional detachment and physical symptoms such
as fatigue, insomnia, headaches, backaches, appetite disruptions, gastrointestinal
alterations and a reduced capacity to function normally in work and personal life
[172]. Burnout is a different but similar concept. It consists of 'feelings of emotional exhaustion, emotional detachment and reduced personal efficacy than can
result from working in a stressful working environment over time' [173, p. 778].

Zadeh, Phillips, Aizvera and Wiener [174] included a list of symptoms
to identify practitioners experiencing burnout (see Table 8.2). This list of

Table 8.2 Symptoms of burnout

Symptoms at work	Symptoms outside work
1. I find myself less engaged in my work with patients, work projects or colleagues.	1. I have had work-related bad dreams/nightmares.
2. I feel irritable with colleagues who invest so much (or so little) time with our patients.	2. I have been unable to get something specific to work out of my head.
3. I feel unable to concentrate at work or get through my daily work tasks.	3. I have thought a lot about quitting my job.
4. I feel unsupported by or unappreciated by my co-workers or supervisors.	4. I worry about my own child/family member getting the same disease as my patients.
5. I feel my paycheck is too low for the work I do.	5. I have unwanted thoughts or memories of children I have worked with pop-up in my head.
6. I have difficulty feeling satisfied that I have done a good job for my patients.	6. I have been questioning my competency in doing the work I have been doing.
	7. I have been feeling dread about going to work.

symptoms should be used as a guideline only and not as a diagnosis. As suggested in the original source, endorsing two or more of these symptoms is a suggestion for and assessment of the possible presence of compassion fatigue.

8.6 Rewards and Challenges

Research with practitioners has identified the main barriers and challenges which practitioners can face when working with children, young people and families in oncology settings. These challenges include, for example, parents not wanting to inform children about their cancer diagnosis [5]. Identifying the correct manner to support parents to talk to children about cancer [2, 6], particularly because there is not a single 'correct' way, depends on the specific children and families.

Regarding rewards, Rohan [173] described that healthcare practitioners can experience satisfaction in their work by easing pain and suffering of their patients. Releasing pain and suffering can lead to receiving gratitude from patients and families. Forming close bonds with patients is another source of reward for healthcare practitioners, as they perceive these bonds as a privilege. Other practitioners described being inspired from witnessing strength and resilience in patients and their families. Some practitioners also reported gaining wisdom and perspective from their work including the appreciation for life and close relationships with people that matter to them. Healthcare practitioners, therefore, can experience challenges but also find significant rewards and even be inspired in the work they do every day.

8.7 Organisational Facilitators and Barriers

Research has found that organisations play a crucial role in practitioners' ability and perceived capacity to support children and families experiencing parental cancer. Workplace culture has an impact on practitioners, and organisation with family-focused care approach can be more successful at providing supports for children and family and putting enablers in place for practitioners to successfully achieve the provision of these supports [64]. Some organisations, for example may have child-friendly environments that allow children to visit their ill parent. Organisations which are family-focused may also encourage further training for practitioners in different topics such as engaging and communicating with children of different ages [64].

Professionals who lack the experience of working with children, particularly novice ones, may never acquire the skills and knowledge to properly support children. For this reason, research has emphasised the importance of offering staff training to develop skills and confidence for staff to address the needs of parents and children [158]. Organisations have a crucial role in enabling self-care for oncology healthcare practitioners. Bowling and Damaskos [172] described those organisations should create an institution-wide compassion fatigue programme with a psycho-educational component about the impact of working with patients with cancer, responses, emotions and reactions associated, as well as ways to cope. This programme needs to be supported by an interdisciplinary planning committee (e.g. nursing, psychiatry, social work, psychology, chaplaincy, human resources, etc.). Research has emphasised the need for multidisciplinary teams to effectively identify and manage the needs of children and young people [158]. Collaborative efforts between parents, teachers and clinicians have also been identified as crucial in supporting young people and ensuring their access to supports [159, 162]. Institutions should also design goals and objectives that fit an institution-wide programme [172]. Overall, the role of organisations is significant, and it requires resources to provide ideal, quality care, but it might also require decision-making and consensus from different voices and disciplines. I understand this might be hard, particularly at first, but it is worth doing for children and families.

Effective record keeping is another important aspect of support provision. If organisations lack formal mechanisms to capture patients' family structures and composition, it may mean that family members, including children and young people become 'invisible' to the system and support provision is more difficult or impossible [158]. This is also why organisational supports are important.

8.8 Policy

Supporting children and families also has significant implications at policy level [64]. The lack of policy available (in most countries as described in Chapter 4) means that the crucial role that practitioners have in supporting parents and their children may be unnoticed and, therefore, not validated. More awareness around these issues needs to be raised to motivate the development of policy and interventions that will help professionals to support ill parents, children and young people [64]. Studies have found that even in the case where policies and procedures were in place to enable the visibility of children in the healthcare system, children's support needs were often overlooked [64].

8.9 Self-Care Strategies

Research has identified that peers can be an important source of reassurance and support for practitioners supporting children and families. Peers can be a source of reassurance, validation and reflection, as well as provide a space to share and debrief with more experienced colleagues regarding the intense emotions experienced in their support role [64, 173].

Healthcare practitioners may benefit from increasing their sources of support including formal supports such as counselling and informal sources such as friends and family, willing to talk, listen, spend time together or do fun and relaxing activities together.

There are several self-care activities that you can try to find out if you like them and if they contribute to your self-care [173, 175]:

- Mindfulness.
- Meditation.
- Journaling.
- Music therapy.
- Breathing exercises.
- Self-awareness.
- Exercise (walking, running, swimming, dancing).
- Hobbies (knitting, reading, listening to music).
- Spiritual practices and other rituals (prayer, meditation).
- Adjusting success expectations (e.g. curing the patient may not be possible, having a dignified death can be the correct option).
- Making meaning (this means finding purpose in the work which justifies the 'cost of caring').
- Physical health medical check-ups to ensure you are physically fit and well.

8.10 Create a Self-Care Plan

Self-care plans have been recommended for healthcare workers [176]. Self-care plans can help health practitioners recognise their personal stressors, emotional states both at work and in their daily life. The following techniques might support your self-care, and it is important to find out what works for you [171, 176].

1. **Knowledge.** Having more knowledge can make you feel more confident and prepared in your role. Attending courses, briefings and trainings that will support you in this can help.

2. **Health**. Your physical and emotional health are crucial to be able to carry out your work. Make sure you are eating nutritious food, taking enough rest and are properly hydrated.

3. **Boundaries**. Setting boundaries for yourself might be helpful, for example limiting shift lengths, the number of patients you see in a day.

4. **Media**. Limit your exposure to media or social media, particularly bad and sad news.

5. **Emotions**. Pay attention to your emotions during your work and take the time to reflect on these emotions and how they are impacting your work.

6. **Release emotion**. Find healthy ways to release emotion when you need it. This might include talking to someone, exercising, journaling, artistic expressions, etc.

7. **Social supports**. Contact friends and family regularly or if you need professional help seek it.

8. **Buddy system**. You can team up with another colleague to take care of each other and to check with each other regularly.

Big Squeeze [177]

Close your eyes and be very still. First of all, squeeze your fists as tight as you can. See if you can make each fist into a tiny ball. How tiny can you make your fists? Now uncurl your fingers very, very slowly, and relax your hands. Let them drop down and become heavy. Now squeeze your arms very tightly against your body. Squeeze, squeeze, squeeze then relax and let them become heavy. And now squeeze your shoulders right up to your ears, squeeze, and squeeze, and let them drop down again and relax. Squeeze your face into a tiny knot, squeeze, and squeeze. Squeeze your eyes very tight, squeeze your nose, squeeze your mouth together, squeeze your cheeks, and now let them go and relax, relax, relax. Pull in your tummy and bottom as tight as you can, squeeze and squeeze and squeeze, then let them go, and relax again. Now squeeze your legs together as much as you can squeeze and squeeze, and then relax them again. Squeeze your feet as tight as you can, squeeze and squeeze and squeeze, and then relax them again. You should be feeling very relaxed now. Just stay here for a while and enjoy this feeling of deep relaxation. Take in a deep breath and as you breathe in say to yourself, *I am relaxed, I am relaxed, I am relaxed*. Breathe out and say to yourself *I am relaxed, I am relaxed, I am relaxed*.

And now, when you are ready, wiggle your fingers and toes, have a big stretch, and open your eyes.

I AM RELAXED, I AM RELAXED (p. 27)

8.11 Implications for Practice

- Appropriate supports should be available for practitioners working with children and families, particularly in the cases of loss and bereavement [162].

- Develop mechanisms that facilitate effective communication (and networking) with practitioners involved in the support of children and families [162]. This will enable mutual support and facilitate consultation and debriefing (if relevant).

- Organisations/hospitals should be engaged to effectively support staff and incentivise self-care.

- Self-care strategies counter experiences that generate stress (compassion fatigue, burnout) as well as opportunities to explore coping and self-care (resilience).

Long Stretch [177]

Close your eyes and be very still. You are going to do an exercise to really feel your muscles stretching and then relaxing. Start with the face. Can you open your eyes wide, and now your nose and mouth? Can you open your ears wide? Stretch your whole face as much as you can. Stretch and stretch and now relax, relax, relax. Now stretch your neck as far as you can. Stretch, stretch, stretch, and relax, relax, relax. And now stretch your back. Feel your whole spine stretching up. Stretch, stretch, stretch, and relax, relax, relax. Feel your chest and tummy stretching. Stretch, stretch, stretch and relax, relax, relax. Stretch your arms far away from your body. Feel the muscles in your arms getting longer as you stretch. Stretch, stretch, stretch, and relax, relax, relax. Stretch your fingers. How long can you make them stretch, stretch, stretch, and relax, relax, relax. Now stretch your legs. Stretch, stretch, stretch, relax, relax, relax. And finally, your feet. Stretch your toes as far as you can. Stretch, stretch, stretch, and relax, relax, relax.

And now, when you are ready, wiggle your fingers and toes, have a big stretch, and open your eyes.

MY BODY FEELS OPEN AND RELAXED,
MY BODY FEELS OPEN AND RELAXED

8.12 Measures

The following is a diagnostic tool that I encourage you to not use as such, unless it is part of a supportive process with a professional that can support you fully. The list of symptoms can help you identify potential issues that you may have experienced or are currently experiencing and this will help you identify if you might have some indication of burnout or compassion fatigue or you might be tired, fatigued or require to take care of yourself a little bit (so please do!).

ProQOL

This tool is used to measure negative and positive affect in relation to helping others who experience suffering and trauma [178]. This tool has specific sub-scales to measure compassion satisfaction, burnout and compassion fatigue.

ProQOL is available in English and over 25 more languages. It is currently a free tool available at https://proqol.org/proqol-measure if the author is credited, it is not altered (except the terms in square brackets) and it is not sold.

Professional Quality of Life Scale (ProQOL)

Compassion Satisfaction and Compassion Fatigue
(ProQOL) Version 5 (2009)

When you *[help]* people you have direct contact with their lives. As you may have found, your compassion for those you *[help]* can affect you in positive and negative ways. Below are some-questions about your experiences, both positive and negative, as a *[helper]*. Consider each of the following questions about you and your current work situation. Select the number that honestly reflects how frequently you experienced these things in the *last 30 days*.

I=Never	2=Rarely	3=Sometimes	4=Often	5=Very Often

_____ 1. I am happy.

_____ 2. I am preoccupied with more than one person I *[help]*.

_____ 3. I get satisfaction from being able to *[help]* people.

_____ 4. I feel connected to others.

_____ 5. I jump or am startled by unexpected sounds.

_____ 6. I feel invigorated after working with those I *[help]*.

_____ 7. I find it difficult to separate my personal life from my life as a *[helper]*.

_____ 8. I am not as productive at work because I am losing sleep over traumatic experiences of a person I *[help]*.

_____ 9. I think that I might have been affected by the traumatic stress of those I *[help]*.

_____ 10. I feel trapped by my job as a *[helper]*.

_____ 11. Because of my *[helping]*, I have felt "on edge" about various things.

_____ 12. I like my work as a *[helper]*.

_____ 13. I feel depressed because of the traumatic experiences of the people I *[help]*.

_____ 14. I feel as though I am experiencing the trauma of someone I have *[helped]*.

_____ 15. I have beliefs that sustain me.

_____ 16. I am pleased with how I am able to keep up with *[helping]* techniques and protocols.

_____ 17. I am the person I always wanted to be.

_____ 18. My work makes me feel satisfied.

_____ 19. I feel worn out because of my work as a *[helper]*.

_____ 20. I have happy thoughts and feelings about those I *[help]* and how I could help them.

_____ 21. I feel overwhelmed because my case [work] load seems endless.

_____ 22. I believe I can make a difference through my work.

_____ 23. I avoid certain activities or situations because they remind me of frightening experiences of the people I *[help]*.

_____ 24. I am proud of what I can do to *[help]*.

_____ 25. As a result of my *[helping]*, I have intrusive, frightening thoughts.

_____ 26. I feel "bogged down" by the system.

_____ 27. I have thoughts that I am a "success" as a *[helper]*.

_____ 28. I can't recall important parts of my work with trauma victims.

_____ 29. I am a very caring person.

_____ 30. I am happy that I chose to do this work.

Professional Quality of Life Scale (ProQOL): A tool to identify compassion fatigue.

References

[1] L. Behar. Interventions with parental cancer, dependent children, and adolescents. In: Christ G., Messner C. and Behar L., eds. *Handbook of oncology social work: Psychosocial care for people with cancer*. Oxford University Press, 2015; 417–418.

[2] A. Arber. How do nurses 'think family' and support parents diagnosed with cancer who have dependent children? *Asia-Pacific Journal of Oncology Nursing*, 2016, 3(3): 214–217.

[3] A. Walczak, F. McDonald, P. Patterson et al. How does parental cancer affect adolescent and young adult offspring? A systematic review. *International Journal of Nursing Studies*, 2018, 77: 54–80. http://doi.org/10.1016/j .ijnurstu.2017.08.017

[4] R. Fearnley. Supporting children when a parent has a life-threatening illness: The role of the community practitioner. *Community Practitioner*, 2012, 85(12): 22–25.

[5] C. Semple and E. McCaughan. Developing and testing a theory-driven e-learning intervention to equip healthcare professionals to communicate with parents impacted by parental cancer. *European Journal of Cancer Care*, 2019, 41: 126–134.

[6] R. Fearnley and J. Boland. Communication and support from health-care professionals to families, with dependent children, following the diagnosis of parental life-limiting illness: A systematic review. *Palliative Medicine*, 2017, 31(3): 212–222. http://doi .org/10.1177/0269216316655736

[7] J. Morris, D. Turnbull, A. Martini et al. Coping and its relationship to post-traumatic growth, emotion, and resilience among adolescents and young adults impacted by parental cancer. *Journal of Psychosocial Oncology*, 2019, 38(1): 73–88. http://doi.org/10.1080/0734 7332.2019.1637384

[8] K. Jansson and A. Anderzen-Carlsson. Adolescents' perspectives of living with a parent's cancer: A unique and personal experience. *Cancer Nursing*, 2017, 40(2): 94–101. http://doi.org/10.1097/ NCC.0000000000000358

[9] L. Kristjanson, K. Chalmers and R. Woodgate. Information and support needs of adolescent children of women with breast cancer. *Oncology Nursing Forum*, 2004, 31(1): 111–119.

[10] R. Lally, J. Hydeman, C. Brooks et al. Experiences and needs of African American children and adolescents in supportive care roles for a relative with breast cancer. *Oncology Nursing Forum*, 2020, 47(2): 165–176. http://doi .org/10.1188/20.ONF.165-176

[11] E. Karlsson, K. Andersson and B. Ahlstrom. Loneliness despite the presence of others – Adolescents' experiences of having a parent who becomes ill with cancer.

European Journal of Oncology Nursing, 2013, **17**(6): 697–703. http://doi.org/10.1016/j.ejon.2013.09.005

[12] C. Hailey, J. Yopp, A. Deal et al. Communication with children about a parent's advanced cancer and measures of parental anxiety and depression: A cross-sectional mixed-methods study. *Support Care Cancer*, 2018, **26**(1): 287–295.

[13] J. Rolland. Cancer and the family: An integrative model. *Cancer Supplement*, 2005, **104**(11): 2584–2595. http://doi.org/10.1002/cncr.21489

[14] A. Visser, G. Huizinga, W. van der Graaf et al. The impact of parental cancer on children and the family: A review of the literature. *Cancer Treatment Reviews*, 2004, **30**(8): 683–694. http://doi.org/10.1016/j.ctrv.2004.06.001

[15] G. Huizinga, A. Visser, W. Van der Graaf et al. Family-oriented multilevel study on the psychological functioning of adolescent children having a mother with cancer. *Psycho-Oncology*, 2011, **20**(7): 730–737. http://doi.org/10.1002/pon.1779

[16] J. Chin and M. Lin. Children's experiences of living with maternal breast cancer: A qualitative study. *Journal of Advanced Nursing*, 2021, **77**(8): 3446–3457. http://doi.org/10.1111/jan.14866

[17] C. O'Neill, C. O'Neill and C. Semple. *Children of parents with cancer: An evaluation of psychosocial intervention.* University College Dublin, 2018. http://doras.dcu.ie/22629/1/Final%20Report%20on%20Evaluation%20of%20CLIMB.pdf

[18] F. Kuhne, M. Haagen, C. Baldus et al. Implementation of preventive mental health services for children of physically ill parents: Experiences in seven European countries and health care systems. *General Hospital Psychiatry*, 2013, **35**(2): 147–153. http://doi.org/10.1016/j.genhosppsych.2012.10.005

[19] B. Leedham and B. Meyerowitz. Responses to parental cancer: A clinical perspective. *Journal of Clinical Psychology in Medical Settings*, 1999, **6**(4): 441–461.

[20] C. Semple and E. McCaughan. Family life when a parent is diagnosed with cancer: Impact of a psychosocial intervention for young children. *European Journal of Cancer Care*, 2013, **22**(2): 219–231.

[21] H. Altun, N. Kurtul, A. Arici and E. Yazar. Evaluation of emotional and behavioural problems in school-age children of patients with breast cancer. *Turkish Journal of Oncology*, 2019, **34**(1): 12–20. http://doi.org/10.5505/tjo.2018.1824

[22] B. Lindqvist, F. Schmitt, P. Santalahti et al. Factors associated with the mental health of adolescents when a parent has cancer. *Scandinavian Journal of Psychology*, 2007, **48**(4): 345–351. http://doi.org/10.1111/j.1467-9450.2007.00573.x

[23] A. Welch, M. Wadsworth and B. Compas. Adjustment of children and adolescents to parental cancer. *American Cancer Society*, 1996, **77**(7): 1409–1418.

[24] M. Watson, I. St James-Roberts, S. Ashely et al. Factors associated with emotional and behavioural

problems among school age children of breast cancer patients. *British Journal of Cancer*, 2006, **94**(1): 43–50. http://doi.org/10.1038/sj.bjc.6602887

[25] F. McDonald, P. Patterson, K. White et al. Correlates of unmet needs and psychological distress in adolescent and young adults who have a parent diagnosed with cancer. *Psycho-Oncology*, 2016, **25**(4): 447–454. http://doi.org/10.1002/pon.3942

[26] T. Krattenmacher, F. Kuhne, J. Ernst et al. Parental cancer: Factors associated with children's psychosocial adjustment – A systematic review. *Journal of Psychosomatic Research*, 2012, **72**(5): 344–356. http://doi.org/10.1016/j.jpsychores.2012.01.011

[27] A. Hauskov Graungaard, C. Bendixen, O. Haavet et al. (2017) Somatic symptoms in children who have a parent with cancer: A systematic review. *Clinical Care Health Development*, 2017, **45**(2): 147–158. http://doi.org/10.1111/cch.12647

[28] T. Osborn. The psychosocial impact of parental cancer on children and adolescents: A systematic review. *Psycho-Oncology*, 2007, **16**(2): 101–126. http://doi.org/10.1002/pon.1113

[29] F. Philips. Adolescents living with a parent with advanced cancer: A review of the literature. *Psycho-Oncology*, 2014, **23**(12): 1323–1339. http://doi.org/10.1002/pon.3570

[30] R. Purc-Stephenson and A. Lyseng. How are the kids holding up? A systematic review and meta-analysis on the psychosocial impact of maternal breast cancer on children. *Cancer Treatment Reviews*, 2016, **49**: 45–56. http://doi.org/10.1016/j.ctrv.2016.07.005

[31] B. Grabiak, C. Bender and K. Puskar. The impact of parental cancer on the adolescent: An analysis of the literature. *Psycho-Oncology*, 2007, **16**(2): 127–137. http://doi.org/10.1002/pon.1083

[32] D. Wellisch, S. Ormseth and A. Arechiga. Evolution and emotional symptoms over time among daughters of patients with breast cancer. *Psychosomatics*, 2015, **56**(5): 504–512. http://doi.org/10.1016/j.psym.2014.07.001

[33] M. Davey, L. Gulish, J. Askew et al. Adolescents coping with mom's breast cancer: Developing family intervention programs. *Journal of Marital and Family Therapy*, 2005, **31**(2): 247–258.

[34] M. Davey, J. Askew and K. Godette. Parent and adolescent responses to non-terminal parental cancer: A retrospective multiple-case pilot study. *Families Systems & Health*, 2003, **21**(3): 245–258.

[35] L. Edwards, M. Watson, I. St. James-Roberts et al. Adolescent's stress responses and psychological functioning when parent has early breast cancer. *Psycho-Oncology*, 2008, **17**(10): 1039–1047. http://doi.org/10.1002/pon.1323

[36] S. Pedersen and T. Revenson. Parental illness, family functioning and adolescent well-being: A family ecology framework to guide research. *Journal of Family Psychology*, 2005, **19**(3): 404–409. http://doi.org/10.1037/0893-3200.19.3.404

[37] P. Patterson, F. McDonald, K. White et al. Levels of unmet needs

and distress amongst adolescents and young adults (AYAs) impacted by familial cancer. *Psycho-Oncology*, 2016, **26**(9): 1285–1292. http://doi.org/10.1002/pon.4421

[38] C. O'Neill, C. O'Neill and C. Semple. Children navigating parental cancer: Outcomes for a psychosocial intervention. *Comprehensive Child and Adolescent Nursing*, 2020, **43**(2): 111–127. http://doi.org/10.1080/24694193.2019.1582727

[39] M. Wong, C. Cavanaugh, J. MacLeamy et al. Posttraumatic growth and adverse long-term effects of parental cancer in children. *American Psychological Association*, 2009, **27**(1): 53–63. http://doi.org/10.1037/a0014771

[40] C. Flahault and S. Sultan. On being a child of an ill parent: A Rorschach investigation of adaptation to parental cancer compared to other illnesses. *Rorschachiana*, 2010, **31**(1): 43–69. http://doi.org/10.1027/1192-5604/a000004

[41] R. Teixeira and M. Pereira. Impact do Cancer Parental no Desenvolvimento Psicologico dos Filhos: Uma Revisao da Literatura. *Psicologia: Reflexao e Critica*, 2011, **24**(3): 513–522.

[42] J. Levesque and D. Maybery. Parental cancer: Catalyst for positive growth and change. *Qualitative Health Research*, 2012, **22**(3): 397–408. http://doi.org/10.1177/1049732311421617

[43] S. Gazendam-Donofrio, H. Hoeskstra, W. van der Graaf et al. Adolescents' emotional reactions to parental cancer: Effect on emotional and behavioural problems. *Journal of Paediatric Psychology*, 2011, **36**(3): 346–359.

[44] K. Kissil, A. Nino, S. Jacobs et al. 'It has been a good growing experience for me': Growth experiences among African American youth coping with parental cancer. *Families, Systems & Health*, 2010, **28**(3): 274–289. http://doi.org/10.1037/a0020001

[45] L. Rodriguez. Understanding adolescent adjustment to maternal cancer: A study of personal experiences and psychological factors that promote adjustment. Unpublished PhD thesis, National University of Ireland Galway, 2016.

[46] L. Rodriguez and P. Dolan. 'It's your turn to step into their shoes': The role of empathy in adolescents experiencing maternal cancer. *Qualitative Research Journal*, 2019, **19**(3): 213–224. http://doi.org/10.1108/QRJ-D-18-00045

[47] J. Barnes, L. Kroll, O. Burke et al. Qualitative interview study of communication between parents and children about maternal breast cancer. *BMJ*, 2000, **173**(6): 385–389.

[48] J. Ernst, V. Beler:ein, G. Romer et al. Use and need for psychosocial support in cancer patients: A population-based sample of patients with minor children. *Cancer*, 2013, **119**(12): 2333–2341. http://doi.org/10.1002/cncr.28021

[49] G. Huizinga, A. Visser, Y. Zelders-Steyn et al. Psychological impact of having a parent with cancer. *European Journal of Cancer*, 2011, **47**(3): S239–246. http://doi.org/10.1016/S0959-8049(11)70170-8

[50] G. Christ. Parental Cancer: Developmentally informed practice guidelines for family consultation and communication.

In: Christ G., Messner C. and Behar L., eds. *Handbook of oncology social work: Psychosocial care for people with cancer*. Oxford University Press, 2015; 419–428.

[51] K. Vannatta, J. Grollman R. Noll et al. Impact of maternal cancer on the peer interactions of children at school. *Psycho-Oncology*, 2008, **17**(3): 252–259. http://doi.org/10.1002/pon.1232

[52] C. Semple and T. McCance. Parent's experience of cancer who have young children: A literature review. *Cancer Nursing*, 2010, **33**(2): 110–118.

[53] S. Hedlund. Introduction to working with families in oncology. In: Christ G., Messner C. and Behar L., eds. *Handbook of oncology social work: Psychosocial care for people with cancer*. Oxford University Press, 2015; 379–384.

[54] F. Faccio, F. Ferrari and G. Pravettoni. When a parent has cancer: How does it impact on children's psychosocial functioning? A systematic review. *European Journal of Cancer Care*, 2018, **27**(6): 1–11. http://doi.org/10.1111/ecc.12895

[55] E. Jeppesen, I. Bjelland, S. Fossa et al. Health-related quality of life in teenagers with a parent with cancer. *European Journal of Oncology Nursing*, 2016, **22**: 46–53. http://doi.org/10.1016/j.ejon.2016.03.004

[56] A. Chan, C. Lomma, H. Chih et al. Psychosocial consequences in offspring of women with breast cancer. *Psycho-Oncology*, 2019, **29**(3): 1–8. http://doi.org/10.1002/pon.5294

[57] G. Landi, A. Duzen, P. Patterson et al. Illness unpredictability and psychosocial adjustment

of adolescent and young adults impacted by parental cancer: The mediating role of unmet needs. *Supportive Care in Cancer*, 2021, **30**(2): 3. http://doi.org/10.1007/s00520-021-06379-3

[58] G. Forrest, C. Plumb, S. Ziebland S. et al. Breast cancer in the family-children's perceptions of their mother's cancer and its initial treatment: Qualitative study. *BMJ*, 2006, **332**(7548): 998–1003. http://doi.org/10.1136/bmj.38793.567801.AE

[59] A. Maynard, P. Patterson, F. McDonald et al. What is helpful to adolescents who have a parent diagnosed with cancer? *Journal of Psychosocial Oncology*, 2013, **31**(6): 675–697. http://doi.org/10.1080/07347332.2013.835021

[60] K. Chalmers, L. Kristjanson, R. Woodgate et al. Perceptions of the role of the school in providing information and support to adolescent children of women with breast cancer. *Journal of Advanced Nursing*, 2000, **31**(6): 1430–1438.

[61] M. Azarbarzin, A. Malekian and F. Taleghani. Adolescents' experiences when living with a parent with cancer: A qualitative study. *Iranian Red Crescent Medical Journal*, 2016, **18**(1): e26410. http://doi.org/10.5812/ircmj.26410

[62] M. Aasebo Hauken, A. Dyregrov and M. Senneseth. Characteristics of the social networks of families living with parental cancer and support provided. *Journal of Clinical Nursing*, 2019, **28** (15–16): 3021–3032. http://doi.org/10.1111/jocn.14859

[63] M. Viegas. *How to be happy*. UK: Our Street Books, 2014.

[64] P. Franklin, A. Arber, L. Reed et al. Health and social care

professional's experiences of supporting parents and their dependent children during, and following, the death of a parent: A qualitative review and thematic synthesis. *Palliative Medicine*, 2019, **33**(1): 49–65. http://doi.org/10.1177/0269216318803494

[65] J. Puterman and S. Cadell. Timing is everything. *Journal of Psychosocial Oncology*, 2008, **26**(2): 103–121. http://doi.org/10.1300/j077v26n02_07

[66] E. Garrad, K. Fennell and C. Wilson. 'We're completely back to normal, but I'd say it's a new normal': A qualitative exploration of adaptive functioning in rural families following a parental cancer diagnosis. *Support Care Cancer*, 2017, **25**(11): 3561–3568. http://doi.org/10.1007/s00520-017-3785-6

[67] Y. Rodriguez-Loyola and R. Costas-Muniz. El diagnóstico de cáncer de mamas desde una perspectiva familiar: Retos para la psico-oncología en América Latina. *Interamerican Journal of Psychology*, 2013, **47**(1): 121–130.

[68] J. Turner. Children's and family needs of young women with advanced breast cancer: A review. *Palliative and Supportive Care*, 2004, **2**(1): 55–64. http://doi.org/10.1017/S1478951504040076

[69] J. Morris, A. Martini and D. Preen. The well-being of children impacted by a parent with cancer: An integrative review. *Support Care Cancer*, 2016, **24**(7): 3235–3251. http://doi.org/10.1007/s00520-016-3214-2

[70] J. Bultmann, V. Beierlein, G. Romer et al. Parental cancer: Health-related quality of life and current psychosocial support needs of cancer survivors and their children. *International Journal of Cancer*, 2014, **135**(11): 2668–2677. http://doi.org/10.1002/ijc.28905

[71] M. Niemela, R. Paananen, H. Hakko et al. Mental disorder diagnoses of offspring affected by parental cancer before early adulthood: The 1987 Finnish Birth Control study. *Psycho-Oncology*, 2016, **25**(12): 1477–1484. http://doi.org/10.1002/pon.4088

[72] H. Gotze, J. Ernst, E. Brahler et al. Predictors of quality of life of cancer patients, their children, and partners. *Psycho-Oncology*, 2015, **24**(7): 787–795. http://doi.org/10.1002/pon.3725

[73] K. Krauel, A. Simon, N. Krause-Hebecker et al. When a parent has cancer: Challenges to patients, their families and health providers. *Expert Review of Pharmacoeconomics & Outcomes Research*, 2012, **12**(6): 795–808. http://doi.org/10.1586/erp.12.62

[74] S. Helseth and N. Ulfsaet. Parenting experiences during cancer. *Journal of Advanced Nursing*, 2005, 52(1): 38–46. http://doi.org/10.1111/j.1365-2648.2005.03562.x

[75] C. Marshall, L. Larkey, M. Curran et al. Considerations of culture and social class for families facing cancer: The need for a new model for health promotion and psychosocial intervention. *Family Systems Health*, 2011, **29**(2): 81–94. http://doi.org/10.1037/a0023975

[76] F. Schmitt, P. Santalahti, S. Saarelainen et al. Cancer families with children: Factors associated with family functioning – A comparative study in Finland. *Psycho-Oncology*, 2008, **17**(4): 363–372. http://doi.org/10.1002/pon.124

[77] K. Stefanou, E. Zografos, Zografos G., et al. Emotional and behavioural problems in children dealing with maternal breast cancer: A literature review. *British Journal of Guidance & Counselling*, 2020, **48**(3), 394–406. http://doi.org/10.1080/03069885.2018.1487530

[78] F. Lewis. The Impact of Breast Cancer on Adolescent Function. 2007. (15) (PDF) The Impact of Breast Cancer on Adolescent Function (researchgate.net)

[79] M. Buchbinder, J. Loghofer and K. McCue. Family routines and rituals when a parent has cancer. *Families, Systems & Health*, 2009, **27**(3), 213–227. http://doi.org/10.1037/a0017005

[80] F. Walsh. Family resilience: A framework for clinical practice. *Family Process*, 2003, **42**(1): 1–18. http://doi.org/10.1111/j.1545-5300.2003.00001.x

[81] E. Alexander, M. O'Connor, C. Rees and G. Halkett. A systematic review of the current interventions available to support children living with parental cancer. *Patient Education and Counselling*, 2019, **102**(10): 1812–1821. http://doi.org/10.1016/j.pec.2019.05.001

[82] S. Gazendam-Donofrio, H. Hoekstra, W. van der Graaf et al. Parent-child communication patterns during the first year after a parent's cancer diagnosis. *Cancer*, 2009, **115**(18): 4227–4237. http://doi.org/10.002/cncr.24502

[83] M. Shands and M. Lewis. Parents with advanced cancer: Worries about their children's unspoken concerns. *American Journal of Hospice and Palliative Medicine*, 2020, **38**(8): 920–926. http://doi.org/10.1177/1049909120969120

[84] L. Sheperd. Developmental strategies for counselling the child whose parent or sibling has cancer. *Journal of Counselling and Development*, 1997, **75**(6): 417–427.

[85] R. Tavares, T. Brandao and P. Matos. Mothers with breast cancer: A mixed-method systematic review on the impact on parent-child relationship. *Psycho-Oncology*, 2016, **27**(2): 367–375. http://doi.org/10.1002/pon.4451

[86] L. Behar and Marcus Lewis. Single parents coping with cancer and children. In: Christ G., Messner C. and Behar L., eds. *Handbook of oncology social work: Psychosocial care for people with cancer*. Oxford University Press, 2015; 429–434.

[87] J. Morris, J. Ohan and A. Martini. An investigation of support services available by Internet searching to families impacted by a parent's cancer. *Psycho-Oncology*, 2018, **27**(1): 114–124. http://doi.org/10.1002/pon.4478

[88] J. Matuszczak-Swigon and L. Bakiera. Experiences of adults as parents with cancer: A systematic review and thematic synthesis of qualitative studies. *Journal of Psychosocial Oncology*, 2021, **39**(6): 765–788. http://doi.org/10.1080/07347332.2020.1859662

[89] K. Weaver, J. Rowland, C. Alfano et al. Parental cancer and the family: A population-based estimate of the number of US Cancer survivors residing with the minor children. *Cancer*, 2010, **116**(18): 4395–4401. http://doi.org/10.1002/cncr.25368

[90] C. O'Neill, E. McCaughan C. Semple et al. Fatherhood and cancer: A commentary on the literature. *European Journal of Cancer Care*, 2013, **22**(2): 161–168. http://doi.org/10.1111/ecc.12021

[91] C. Rashi, T. Wittman, A. Tsimicalis et al. Balancing illness and parental demands: Coping with cancer while raising minor children. *Oncology Nursing Forum*, 2015, **42**(4): 337–344.

[92] E. Elmberger, C. Bolund and K. Lutzen. Experience of dealing with moral responsibility as a mother with cancer. *Nursing Ethics*, 2005, **12**(3):253–262. http://doi .org/10.1191/0969733005ne787oa

[93] J. Christine, V. Beierlein, G. Romer et al. Use and need for psychosocial support in cancer patients. *Cancer*, 2013, **119**(2): 2333–2341. http://doi.org/10.1002/ cncr.28021

[94] A. Dezinger, M. Bingisser, V. Ehrbar et al. Web-based counselling for families with parental cancer: Baseline findings and lessons learned. *Journal of Psychosocial Oncology*, 2019, **37**(5): 599–615. http://doi.org/10.1080/07 347332.2019.1602576

[95] Y. Colon. Sociocultural and economic diversity: Improving access and health outcomes. In: Christ G., Messner C. and Behar L., eds. *Handbook of oncology social work: Psychosocial care for people with cancer*. Oxford University Press, 2015; 261–263.

[96] Y. Colon. Working with sociocultural and economic diversity. In: Christ G., Messner C. and Behar L., eds. *Handbook of oncology social work: Psychosocial care for people with cancer*. Oxford University Press, 2015; 263–268.

[97] H. Freeman. Poverty, culture and social injustice: Determinants of cancer disparities. *CA Cancer Journal for Clinicians*, 2004, **54**(2): 72–77.

[98] J. Morris, I. Zajac, D. Turnbull et al. A longitudinal investigation of Western Australia families impacted by parental cancer with adolescent and young adult offspring. *Australian and New Zealand Journal of Public Health*, 2019, **43**(3): 261–266. http://doi .org/10.1111/1753-6405.12885

[99] M. Davey, C. Tubbs, K. Kissil and A. Nino. 'We are survivors too': African-American youths' experiences of coping with parental breast cancer. *Psycho-Oncology*, 2011, **20**(1): 77–87. http://doi.org/10.1002/pon.1712

[100] A. Amodio and U. Roy. Support for immigrants, political refugees, and patients seeking asylum who have cancer. In: Christ G., Messner C. and Behar L., eds. *Handbook of oncology social work: Psychosocial care for people with cancer*. Oxford University Press, 2015; 269–274.

[101] F. Phillips, E. Prezio, L. Panisch & B. Jones. Factors affecting outcomes following a psychosocial intervention for children when a parent has cancer. *The Journal of Child Life: Psychosocial Theory and Practice*, 2021, **2**(2): 1–13.

[102] A. Martini, J. Morris, H. Jackson et al. The impact of parental cancer on preadolescent children (0–11 years) in Western Australia: A longitudinal population study. *Supportive Care in Cancer*, 2019, **27**(4): 1229–1236. http://doi .org/10.1007/s00520-018-4480-y

[103] P. Pui-Yu and C. L. Chan. Working with Chinese families impacted by cancer: An integrative body-mind-spirit approach. In: Christ G., Messner C. and Behar L., eds. *Handbook of oncology social work: Psychosocial care for people with*

cancer. Oxford University Press, 2015; 305–310.

[104] M. Ghofrani, L. Nikfarid, M. Nourian et al. Levels of unmet needs among adolescents and young adults (AYAs) impacted by parental cancer. *Supportive Care in Cancer*, 2019, **27**(1): 175–182. http://doi .org/10.1007/s00520-018-4310-2

[105] C. Reyes, R. Palacios, K. Sondgeroth et al. Young child-rearing Latina cancer survivors living in the US-Mexico border region: A qualitative study. *Journal of Cancer Therapy*, 2021, **12**(4): 174–185. http://doi.org/10.4236/ jct.2021.124018

[106] R. Costas-Muniz. Hispanic adolescents coping with parental cancer. *Support Care Cancer*, 2012, **20**(2): 413–417. http://doi .org/10.1007/s00520-011-1283-9

[107] A. Marin-Chollom. Latino/a adolescents and young adults coping with parental cancer within a cultural context. Unpublished PhD thesis, The City University of New York, 2017.

[108] H. Ainuddin, S. Loh, W. Low, et al. Quality of life of multi-ethnic adolescents living with a parent with cancer. *Asian Pacific Journal of Cancer Prevention*, 2012, **13**(12): 6289–6294. http://doi.org/10.7314/ APjcp.2012.13.12.6289

[109] S. Mat Saat, M. Hepworth and T. Jackson. 'She looked like and Alien': Experience and definitions children attach to a cancer diagnosis. *Aslib Journal of Information Management*, 2018, **70**(1): 78–103. http://doi .org/10.1108/AJIM-06-2017-0142

[110] K. Bullock and H. Allison. Access to medical treatment for African Americans diagnosed with cancer:

The current evidence base. In: Christ G., Messner C. and Behar L., eds. *Handbook of oncology social work: Psychosocial care for people with cancer*. Oxford University Press, 2015; 293–297.

[111] Halso-och Sjukvårdslag (SFS 2017:13) Stockholm: Socialdepartementet. www.riksdagen.se/sv/ dokument-lagar/dokument/ svensk-forfattningssamling/ halsooch-sjukvardslag_sfs-2017-30

[112] S. Knutsson, K. Enskar and M. Golsater Nurses' experiences of what constitutes the encounter with children visiting a sick parent at an adult ICU. *Intensive and Critical Care Nursing*, 2017, **39**: 9–17. http:// doi.org/10.1016/j.iccn.2016.09.003

[113] A. Syse, G. Aas and J. Loge. Children and young adults with parents with cancer: A population-based study. *Clinical Epidemiology*, 2012, **4**: 41–52. http://doi .org/10.2147/CLEP.S28984

[114] F. Al-Zaben, S. Al-Amoudi, B. El-deek and H. Koenig. Impact of maternal breast cancer on school-aged children in Saudi Arabia. *BMC Research Notes*, 2014, **7**: 261–265. http://doi .org/10.1186/1756-0500-7-261

[115] W. Chang. Will my disclosure harm the relationship? Factors that impact mother-daughter cancer communication in Taiwan. *American Journal of Qualitative Research*, 2021, **5**(2): 171–189. http://doi.org/10.29333/ajqr/11241

[116] S. Korbi, Y. Berrazega, M. Nesrine et al. Tunisian children and adolescents coping with parental cancer. *Annals of Oncology*, 2021, **32**(S5). http://doi.org/10.1016/j .annonc.2021.08.817

[117] I. Inoue, T. Higashi, M. Iwato et al. A national profile of the impact of parental cancer on their children in Japan. *Cancer Epidemiology*, 2015, 39(6): 838–841. http://doi.org/10.1016/j.canep.2015.10.005

[118] M. Niemela, R. Paananen, H. Hakko et al. The prevalence of children affected by parental cancer and their use of specialized psychiatric services: The 1987 Finnish Birth Cohort study. *International Journal of Cancer*, 2012, **131**(9): 2177–2125. http://doi.org/10.1002/ijc.27466

[119] M. Franklin, P. Patterson, K. Allison et al. An invisible patient: Healthcare professional's perspectives on caring for adolescents and young adults who have a sibling with cancer. *European Journal of Cancer Care*, 2018, **27**(6): e12970. http://doi.org/10.1111/ecc.12970

[120] N. Weeks, F. McDonald, P. Patterson et al. A summary of high-quality online information resources for parents with cancer who have adolescent and young adult children: A scoping review. *Psycho-Oncology*, 2019, 28(12): 2323–2335. http://doi.org/10.1002/pon.5274

[121] S. Jorgensen, L. Thygesen, S. Michelsen, P. Due et al. Why do some adolescents manage despite parental illness? Identifying promoting factors. *Journal of Adolescent Health*, 2021, 69(2): 335–341. http://doi.org/10.1016/j.adohealth.2020.12.139

[122] Cancer.Net. Talking with Children about Cancer. 2019. www.cancer.net/coping-with-cancer/talking-with-family-and-friends/talking-about-cancer/talking-with-children-about-cancer

[123] Irish Cancer Society. Talking to Children about Cancer. 2017. www.cancer.ie/cancer-information-and-support/cancer-support/coping-with-cancer/information-for-patients/talking-to-family-and-friends

[124] MacMillan Cancer Support. Talking to children and teenagers when an adult has cancer. 2019. cdn.macmillan.org.uk/dfsmedia/1a6f23537f7f4519b b0cf14c45b2a629/803-source/talking-to-children-and-teenagers-when-an-adult-has-cancer-mac5766-e04-n?_ga=2.145 805300.198515011.1631459 114-1955156953.1631459114

[125] V. Kazlauskaite and S. Fife. Adolescent experience with parental cancer and involvement with medical professionals: A heuristic phenomenological inquiry. *Journal of Adolescent Research*, 2021, **36**(4):1–28. http://doi.org/10.1177/0743558420985446

[126] World Health Organization. Cancer. 2021. www.who.int/news-room/fact-sheets/detail/cancer

[127] National Cancer Institute. Cancer Statistics. 2021. www.cancer.gov/about-cancer/understanding/statistics

[128] F. Philips and E. Prezio. Wonders & Worries: Evaluation of a chid centred psychosocial intervention for families who have a parent/primary caregiver with cancer. *Psycho-Oncology*, 2016, **26**(7): 1006–1012. http://doi.org/10.1002/pon.4120

[129] J. Ohan, H. Jackson, S. Bay et al. How psychosocial interventions meet the needs of children of parents with cancer: A review

and critical evaluation. *European Journal of Cancer Care*, 2020, **29**(5): 1–16. http://doi.org/10.1111/ecc.13237

[130] M. Thastum. A. Munch-Hansen, A. Wiell et al. Evaluation of a focused short-term preventive counselling project for families with a parent with cancer. *Clin Child Psychol Psychiatry*, 2006, **11**(4): 529–542. http://doi.org/10.1177/1359104506067875

[131] M. Kobayashi, S. Heiney, Osawa K. et al. Effect of a group intervention for children and their parents who have cancer. *Palliative and Supportive Care*, 2007, **15**(5): 575–586.

[132] L. Northouse, J. Walker, A. Schafenacker et al. A family-based program of care for women with recurrent breast cancer and their family members, *Oncology Nursing Forum*, 2002, **29**(10): 1411–1419.

[133] L. Inhestern, A. Haller, O. Wlodarczyk et al. Psychosocial interventions for families with parental cancer and barriers and facilitators to implementation and use – A Systematic Review. *PLoS One*, 2016, **11**(6): e0156967. http://doi.org/10.1371/journal.pone.0156967

[134] S. J. Eillis, C. E. Wakefiled, G. Antill et al. Supporting children facing a parent's cancer diagnosis: A systematic review of children's psychosocial needs and existing interventions. *European Journal of Cancer Care*, 2017, **26**(1), 1–22. http://doi.org/10.1111/ecc.12432

[135] M. Niemela, H. Hakko and S. Rasanen. A systematic narrative review of the studies on structured child-centred interventions for families with a parent with cancer. *Psycho-Oncology*, 2010, **19**(5): 451–461. http://doi.org/10.1002/pon.1620

[136] L. Northouse. Helping families of patients with cancer. *Oncology Nursing Forum*, 2005, **32**(4): 743–750.

[137] A. Jackson, C. Holmes, J. Looby et al. Therapeutic interventions with families of breast cancer survivors. *Journal of Feminist Family Therapy*, 2021, **33**(1): 40–58. http://doi.org/10.1080/08952833.2021.1872268

[138] M. Dohmen, A. Petermann-Meyer, D. Blei, R. Bremen et al. Comprehensive support for families with parental cancer (Family-SCOUT), evaluation of a complex intervention: Study protocol for a non-randomized controlled trial. *Trials*, 2021, **22**: 1–10. http://doi.org/10.21203/rs.3.rs-401056/v

[139] L. Stafford, M. Sinclair, J. Turner et al. Study protocol for Enhancing Parenting in Cancer (EPIC): Development and evaluation of a brief psycho-educational intervention to support parents with cancer who have young children. *Pilot and Feasibility Studies*, 2017, **3**(72): 1–9. http://doi.org/10.186/s40814-017-0215-y

[140] F. Phillips and E. Prezio. Wonders & Worries: Evaluation of a child centered psychosocial intervention for families who have a parent/primary caregiver with cancer. *Psycho-Oncology*, 2017, **26**(7): 1006–1012. http://doi.org/10.1002/pon.4120

[141] M. Bingisser, D. Eichelberger, V. Ehrbar et al. Web-based counselling for families with parental cancer: A case report.

Psycho-Oncology, 2018, **27**(6): 1667–1669. http://doi.org/10.1002/pon.4679

[142] C. Oja, T. Edbom, A. Nager et al. Informing children of their parent's illness: A systematic review of intervention programs with child outcomes in all health care settings globally from inception to 2019. *PLoS One*, 2020, **15**(5). http://doi.org/10.1371/journal.pone.0233696

[143] K. Nelson. A parallel group program for parents and children: Using expressive techniques and activities to facilitate communication. In: Christ G., Messner C. and Behar L., eds. *Handbook of oncology social work: Psychosocial care for people with cancer.* Oxford University Press, 2015; 435–441.

[144] M. Inada, K. Komatsuzaki, M. Kobayashi et al. Psychosocial support programmes for children who have parents with cancer – Program significance and problems for dissemination in Japan. *Journal of Pain and Symptom Management*, 2016, **52**(6): 92. http://doi.org/10.1016/j.jpainsymman.2016.10.191

[145] L. Inhestern, W. Geertz, F. Schulz-Kindermann et al. Parental cancer: Characteristics of users of child-centred counselling versus individual psycho-oncological treatment. *Psycho-Oncology*, 2018, **27**(3): 955–961. http://doi.org/10.1002/pon.4618

[146] P. Moore, S. Rivera, G. Bravo-Soto et al. Communication skills training for healthcare professionals working with people who have cancer, *Cochrane Database of Systematic Reviews*, 2018, **7**(7).

http://doi.org/10.1002/14651858.CD003751.pub4

[147] D. J. Cegala and S. Lenzmeier Broz. Physician communication skills training: A review of theoretical backgrounds, objectives and skills. *Medical Education*, 2002, **36**(11): 1004–1016.

[148] C. Paul, T. Clinton-McHarg, R. Sanson-Fisher et al. Are we there yet? The state of the evidence base for guidelines on breaking bad news to cancer patients. *European Journal of Cancer*, 2009, **45**(17): 2960–2966.

[149] L. Grant, A. Sangha, S. Lister and T. Wiseman. Cancer and the family: Assessment, communication and brief interventions – The development of an educational programme for healthcare professionals when a parent has cancer. *BMJ Supportive & Palliative Care*, 2016, **6**(4): 493–499. http://doi.org/10.1136/bmjspcare-2015-001006

[150] K. Fasciano, H. Berman, C. Moore et al. When a parent has cancer: A community-based program for school personnel. *Psycho-Oncology*, 2007, **16**(2): 158–167. http://doi.org/10.1002/pon.1148

[151] J. Hanna, E. McCaughan and C. Semple. Challenges and support needs of parents and children when a parent is at end of life: A systematic review. *Palliative Medicine*, 2019, **33**(8): 1017–1044. http://doi.org/10.1177/0269216319857622

[152] C. MacPherson and M. Emeleus. Children's needs when facing the death of a parent from cancer: Part one. *International Journal of Palliative Nursing*, 2007, **13**(12): 590–597.

[153] D. Check, E. Park, K. Reeder-Hayes, et al. Concerns underlying treatment preferences of advanced cancer patients with children. *Psycho-Oncology*, 2017, **26**(10): 1491–1497. http://doi.org/10.1002/pon.4164

[154] K. Bugge, S. Helseth and P. Dabushire. Parent's experiences of a Family Support Program when a parent has incurable cancer. *Journal of Clinical Nursing*, 2009, **18**(24): 3480–3488. http://doi.org/10.1111/j.1365-2702.2009.02871.x

[155] V. Kennedy and M. Lloyd-Williams. How children cope when a parent has advanced cancer. *Psycho-Oncology*, 2009, **18**(8): 886–892. http://doi.org/10.1002/pon.1455

[156] K. Howell, E. Barrett-Becker, A. Burnside et al. Children facing parental cancer versus parental death: The buffering effects of positive parenting and emotional expression. *Journal of Child and Family Studies*, 2016, **25**(1): 152–164. http://doi.org/10.1007/s10826-015-0198-3

[157] J. Kaplow, C. Layne, R. Pynoos et al. DSM-V Diagnostic criteria for bereavement-related disorders in children and adolescents: Developmental considerations. *Psychiatry*, 2012, **75**(3): 243–265.

[158] J. Cockle-Hearne, E. Reed, J. Todd and E. Ream. The dying parent and dependent children: A nationwide survey of hospice and community palliative care support services. *BMJ Supportive & Palliative Care*, 2020. http://doi.org/10.1136/bmjspcare-2019-001947

[159] A. Varathakeyan, F. McDonald, P. Patterson et al. Accessing support before or after a parent dies from cancer and young people's current wellbeing. *Support Care Cancer*, 2018, **26**(3): 797–805. http://doi.org/10.1007/s00520-017-3891-5

[160] C. MacPherson. Difficulties for a practitioner preparing a family for the death of a parent: A narrative inquiry. *Mortality*, 2018, **23**(3): 247–260. http://doi.org/10.1080/13576275.2017.1339677

[161] E. Park, K. Miller and K. Knafl. Understanding familial response to parental advanced cancer using the family management style framework. *Journal of Psychosocial Oncology*, 2019, **37**(6), 758–776. http://doi.org/10.1080/07347332.2019.1614132

[162] C. MacPherson and M. Emeleus. Children's needs when facing the death of a parent from cancer: Part two. *International Journal of Palliative Nursing*, 2007, **13**(10): 478–485.

[163] P. Patterson and A. Rangganadhan. Losing a parent to cancer: A preliminary investigation into the needs of adolescents and young adults. *Palliative and Supportive Care*, 2010, **8**(3): 255–265. http://doi.org/10.1017/S1478951510000052

[164] B. Kramer and A. Boelk. Managing family conflict: Providing responsive family care at the end of life. In: Christ G., Messner C. and Behar L., eds. *Handbook of oncology social work: Psychosocial care for people with cancer*. Oxford University Press, 2015; 399–407.

[165] G. Mireault and B. Compas. A prospective study of coping and adjustment before and after a parent's death from cancer. *Journal*

of Psychosocial Oncology, 1996, **14**(4): 1–18.

[166] Canteen Australia. Now what? Living with the death of your parent, brother or sister from cancer. (n.d.). www.canteen.org.au/wp-content/uploads/2015/07/Living-with-the-death-of-your-parent-or-sibling-from-cancer.pdf

[167] Canteen Australia. A guide to Canteen for school students impacted by cancer. (n.d.). www.canteen.org.au/wp-content/uploads/2020/02/Guide-to-Canteen-for-Schools-2020-version.pdf

[168] F. Kuhne, T. Krattenmacher, C. Bergelt et al. Parental palliative cancer: Psychosocial adjustment and health-related quality of life in adolescents participating in a German family counselling service. *BMC Palliative Care*, 2012, **11**(21): 1–9. www.biomedcentral.com/1472-684X/11/21

[169] R. Moos and B. Moos. *Family Environment Scale Test Manual*. California: Mind Garden, Inc., 1974

[170] M. Golsater, M. Henricson, K. Enskar et al. Are children as relatives our responsibility? How nurses perceive their role in caring for children as relatives of seriously ill patients. *European Journal of Oncology Nursing*, 2016, **25**: 33–39. http://doi.org/10.1016/j.ejon.2016.09.005

[171] S. Sanchez-Reilly, L. Morrison, E. Carey et al. Caring for oneself to care for others: Physicians and their self-care. *The Journal of Supportive Oncology*, 2013, **11**(2): 75–81. http://doi.org/10.12788/j.suponc.0003

[172] J. Bowling and P. Damaskos. Building resilience: A multifaceted support program for professional and support staff in a cancer center. In: Christ G., Messner C. and Behar L., eds. *Handbook of oncology social work: Psychosocial care for people with cancer*. Oxford University Press, 2015; 771–776.

[173] E. Rohan. How oncology professionals manage the emotional intensity of their work. In: Christ G., Messner C. and Behar L., eds. *Handbook of oncology social work: Psychosocial care for people with cancer*. Oxford University Press, 2015; 777–783.

[174] S. Zadeh, J. Phillips, J. Aizvera et al. Maintaining competent teams in paediatric oncology. In: Christ G., Messner C. and Behar L., eds. *Handbook of oncology social work: Psychosocial care for people with cancer*. Oxford University Press, 2015; 801–808.

[175] L. Rodriguez. Propuesta de implementación de una intervención en autocuidado para cuidadoras primarias del "Grupo de madres" de la Asociación Costarricense de Hemofilia: Una intervención desde la Psicología de la Salud. Tesis para optar por el grado de Maestría. Universidad de Costa Rica, 2010.

[176] B. Larkin. Self-care for healthcare workers during disasters. 2016. https://paramedics.org/storage/news/Self-Care%20for%20Healthcare%20workers%20referenced.pdf

[177] M. Viegas. *The Wishing Star. 52 Meditations for Children*. UK: Our Street Books, 2005.

[178] Stamm. The PROQoL Manual. 2002. http://compassionfatigue.org/pages/ProQOLManualOct05.pdf

Index

Printed in the United States
by Baker & Taylor Publisher Services